MUTE WITNESSES

MUTE WITNESSES

TRACE EVIDENCE ANALYSIS

Edited by Max M. Houck

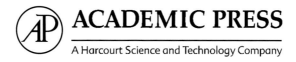

ACADEMIC PRESS

A Harcourt Science and Technology Company

San Diego   San Francisco   New York   Boston
London   Sydney   Tokyo

Copyright © 2001 by ACADEMIC PRESS

ACADEMIC PRESS
A Harcourt Science and Technology Company
Harcourt Place, 32 Jamestown Road, London NW1 7BY, UK
http://www.academicpress.com

ACADEMIC PRESS
A Harcourt Science and Technology Company
525 B Street, Suite 1900, San Diego, California 92101-4495, USA
http://www.academicpress.com

ISBN 0-12-356760-2

Library of Congress Control Number 2001088664
A catalogue record for this book is available from the British Library

Typeset by Kenneth Burnley, Wirral, Cheshire
Printed in Spain by Grafos SA Arte Sobre Papel, Barcelona
01 02 03 04 05 06 GF 9 8 7 6 5 4 3 2 1

CONTENTS

This book is dedicated to
Nicole, Jessica, and Jacqueline.
I wish to God I could have done more for you,
and sooner.

ACKNOWLEDGEMENTS

The authors would like to thank their respective agencies for the time and resources used in the production of this work.

I would like to personally thank Dr Jay Siegel for his guidance and support over the years and for putting me in touch with Nick Fallon of Academic Press. Nick was a prince among men during this project and, despite my best efforts, kept me in line. Carey, Nick needs a raise. Thanks.

I would also like to thank the authors of this book without whom you would be reading something else. I am constantly reminded that giants still walk this Earth: this book is filled with their footprints. What I have learned from working with these scientists has made me a better professional and a better person. If it were not for these dedicated men and women, the gears of Justice would surely lock up and grind to a stop.

The proceeds from the sale of this book go to the Max W. and Janet P. Houck Endowment for the Forensic Sciences at Michigan State University, East Lansing, Michigan. The Endowment is competitive for graduate students seeking a degree in forensic science or forensic anthropology. Thanks, Mom and Dad; I'm still trying.

CONTRIBUTORS

Max M. Houck (Editor)
FBI Laboratory Trace Evidence Unit, Federal Bureau of Investigation, 935 Pennsylvania Avenue NW, Washington, DC 20535, USA.

Ken Wiggins
Forensic Science Service, 109 Lambeth Road, London SE1 7LP, UK.

Douglas W. Deedrick
FBI Laboratory Trace Evidence Unit, Federal Bureau of Investigation, 935 Pennsylvania Avenue NW, Washington, DC 20535, USA.

Susan Ballou
National Institute of Standards and Technology, Office of Law Enforcement Standards, 100 Bureau Drive, Gaithersburg, MD 20899, USA.

Amy Michaud
FBI Laboratory Trace Evidence Unit, Federal Bureau of Investigation, 935 Pennsylvania Avenue NW, Washington, DC 20535, USA.

Brad Putnam
Oregon State Police Crime Laboratory, 3620 Gateway Street, Springfield, OR 97477, USA.

Richard E. Bisbing
McCrone Associates, Inc., 850 Pasquinelli Drive, Westmont, IL 60559, USA.

Scott Ryland
Florida Department of Law Enforcement, 500 W. Robinson Street, Orlando, FL 32801, USA.

José Almirall
Florida International University, Chemistry Department, Miami, FL 33172, USA.

Lee Brun-Conti
Formerly Michigan State Police, Northville Laboratory, 42145 West 7 Mile, Northville, MI 48167, USA, now Bureau of Alcohol, Tobacco and Firearms, Research Boulevard, Rockville, MD.

INTRODUCTION

Ken Wiggins, Forensic Science Service
with Max M. Houck, FBI Laboratory

It was in 1887 that Sir Arthur Conan Doyle first introduced the fictional character Sherlock Holmes. It was through Holmes that Doyle described scientifically based detection methods long before their true value was recognized or they were implemented in "real life" investigations. From these stories, and the various movies and television shows each year, many believe that the life of a forensic scientist is one of glamour, intrigue and excitement. Maybe we should blame, or thank, Doyle for making us spend time convincing others that this really isn't the case. It's amazing how many fictional detectives manage to solve cases within the covers of a book or during a one- or two-hour television program. The recovery, comparison, analysis and interpretation of trace material usually involves many hours, days, weeks or even months of painstaking examinations. This is obviously the point at which fact and fiction differ. The other falsehood that we have to overcome is that many people see us as 'the people who cut up bodies'; yet another myth with which we have to contend because people are watching too much television.

While our discipline has obviously caught the public's imagination, we still struggle to convince detectives, attorneys, and juries of the value of trace evidence. Often characterized as "could have" evidence that only weakly associates the suspect, victim, and the crime scene (because, as the opposing attorney will tell you, "These materials could have come from *anywhere*"), trace evidence is so much more. DNA, despite the public and professional accolades, only answers the question, "Who?" Trace evidence, on the other hand, may be able to tell you "what," "where," "how," and "when."[1] The case reviews that form the text in this book will hopefully do much to set the record straight and to demonstrate the strength and breadth of trace evidence in criminal investigations.

Trace evidence is a generic term for small, often microscopic, fragments of various types of material that transfer between people, places, and objects, and persist there for a time. The range of materials covered by the terminology is enormous and can include fibers, paint, glass, hair, soil, feathers, metal, brick dust, sand, pollen, sawdust and vegetation, to name but a few examples. The focus of most crime scenes is the gross, easily visible evidence: the body, the gun, the blood. Microscopic evidence must not be forgotten, however, simply

[1] I am indebted to Carl Selavka for this phrasing (MMH).

because we cannot see it with the unaided eye. As Paul Kirk noted in his book, *Criminal Investigation*:

> . . . microscopic evidence is present in most cases, and is therefore of much wider availability. If there is a single important lesson to be learned by the investigator, it is the extent to which he may rely on microscopic physical evidence if he is willing to make full use of it (Kirk 1953: 6).

"Full use" in this context means not only proper collection and packaging but also assistance in the identification and timely collection of suitable known samples from relevant sources.

The foundation of trace evidence is contact between people, places, and objects. Typically, the phrase is conceptually limited to small particulate matter but in reality *the majority of forensic evidence is trace evidence*. Blood on a wall, a fingerprint on a knife, gunshot residue deposited around a wound, tire impressions in mud are all evidence of contact between people and/or objects. The lingering evidence is a demonstration of the relationships these people and objects experienced during the commission of the crime and it establishes the context of the crime scene. Physical context is critical to the evidentiary value of forensic results; this is why so much emphasis is placed on crime scene methods in textbooks. Working a crime scene, like excavating an archaeological site, is a process of "careful destruction." Once a piece of evidence is moved or collected, it can never be put back exactly where it was: its provenance is lost for ever. Careful documentation is the essence of a properly processed crime scene and it is through this documentation that the scene is reconstructed in the laboratory.

Social context is just as important, however, and this information is often not communicated properly to the trace analyst. Like the character Pig Pen from the Peanuts cartoon strip, we each carry around with us traces of all our environments with which we interact during our activities. Everyone's environments are different and we transfer bits of these environments in our contacts. The area between the subject of an investigation and the victim changes from probative, if the two are strangers, to less probative, if the two are cohabiting spouses. Trace analysts expect to find an individual's hair in his or her car or on their own clothing. It is the unfamiliar or foreign materials from outside the person's typical environment that are of interest to the trace analyst when examining that person's items. Conversely, a trace analyst is interested in whether or not he finds these same materials on *other people's* items when those are examined. Trace evidence explores the intersections between people's environments and explicates their interactions.

An example may help to illustrate the investigative and confirmatory power of trace evidence. The president of a large multinational oil company left his home for work at 7.30 a.m. At about 8.00 a.m., a neighbor saw the man's unoccupied car with the engine running at the end of the driveway. The local police determined that he did not show up for work that day. As it was a kidnapping with the chance of interstate travel, the FBI took over the investigation.

The victim's family and his company received a number of ransom demands over the course of several weeks; the first, received by the family, demanded $18 million and a cellular phone. The abductors said they were members of an environmentalist group. The FBI felt that because of the recent Exxon Valdez oil spill in Alaska, this type of group might be responsible.

Ransom notes, which had been left at various locations, came in to the FBI with requests for document and fingerprint examinations. It was determined that the items needed to be examined for hairs and fibers first. Several pieces of duct tape attached to the outside of the ransom notes were also examined. Red carpet fibers and dog hairs were found on the first piece of duct tape and on the second piece dog hairs, an 11-inch treated head hair, and gold carpet fibers were found (Figures I.1 through I.4). The trace analyst provided information to the breed of dog and types of cars involved. He also suggested that a female might be involved because of the length and treatment of the head hair found on the tape.

Muffled telephone calls demanding money continued to be received by the victim's family; the FBI determined that were made from phone booths. Agents staked out about 60 phone booths in the area trying to catch the suspects. On 18 June 1992, a man was seen making a call with what appeared to be a tape recorder placed against the receiver at a nearby shopping mall; he was also

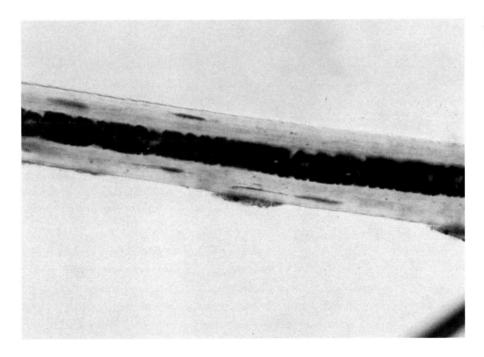

Figure I.1
Questioned dog hairs.

Figure I.2
Questioned fibers.

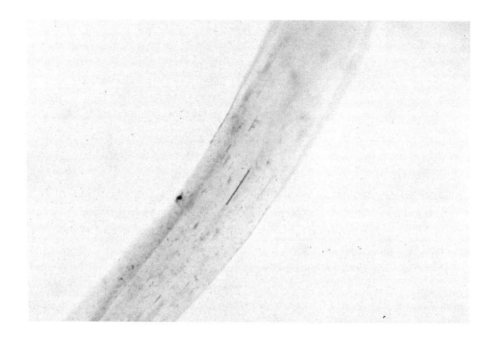

Figure I.3
Questioned fibers.

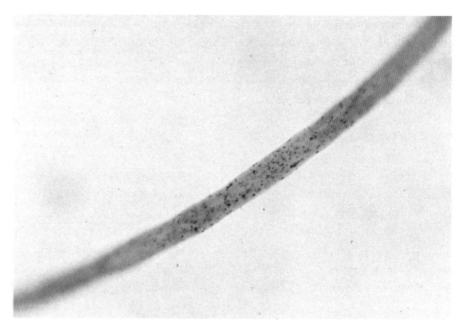

wearing gloves. The suspect got away in a red sedan, but the agents recorded the car's license plate number. The FBI agents ran the tag and discovered it was a rental. They then placed the rental agency under surveillance. When the man returned the car, a red Chevrolet Lumina, they arrested him. His wife came to pick him up a short time later and was also arrested.

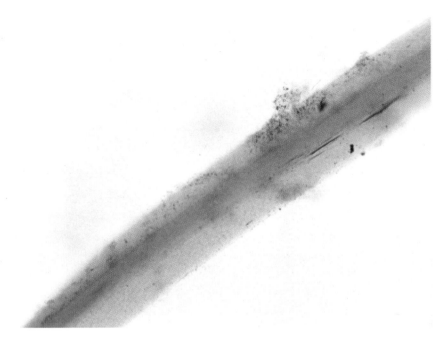

Figure I.4
Questioned red carpet-type fibers

The victim had been taken to a storage facility and kept in a 4′ × 6′ wooden box; the rest of the storage facility was empty. The suspects reportedly gave the victim food and water, but he died while in the box. The suspects buried the body in a remote forested area.

Several searches were conducted at the suspect's residence, the suspect's cars, and a self-storage facility. During the interviews and searches, FBI agents found a one-way airline ticket for the husband but no accompanying ticket for his wife. The agents convinced the wife that her husband was going to take the money and leave her behind. She told the agents everything and took them to the area where the body was buried. The box the victim was kept in was never found.

The rental car was a 1992 Chevrolet Lumina with a red interior and carpets (Figure I.5). The wife was driving a 1984 Mercedes (Figure I.6). The head hair matched the suspect's daughter's hair and the dog hair matched the family's golden retriever (Figure I.7). Other fibers recovered from the duct tape and the ransom notes matched fibers from the car carpets and the suspect's house (Figures I.8 to I.10). The cars were used to transport the ransom demands and instructions. The suspect's wife told the FBI that she had placed the demand notes on the floor of her Mercedes. When confronted with the evidence linking their car, the rental car, their dog, and home environment to the body, the suspects pleaded guilty in Federal Court to extortion and conspiracy; they also pleaded guilty in state court to kidnapping and felony murder.

Figure I.5

The interior of the 1992 red Chevrolet Lumina rental car.

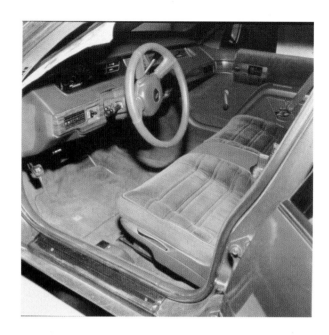

Figure I.6

The interior of the white 1984 Mercedes.

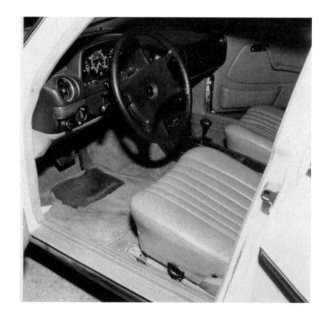

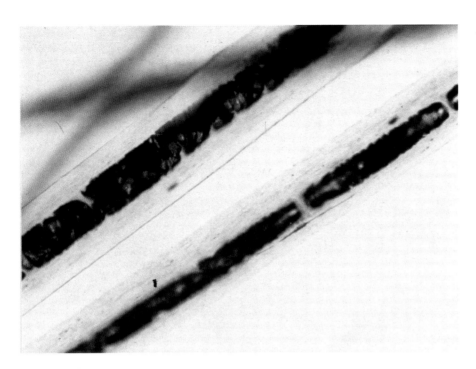

Figure I.7
Known hairs from the
suspect's golden retriever.

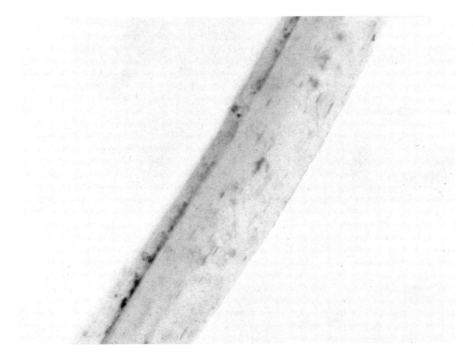

Figure I.8
Fibers from the 1984
Mercedes floor mats.

Figure I.9

*Known fibers from the
1984 Mercedes carpeting.*

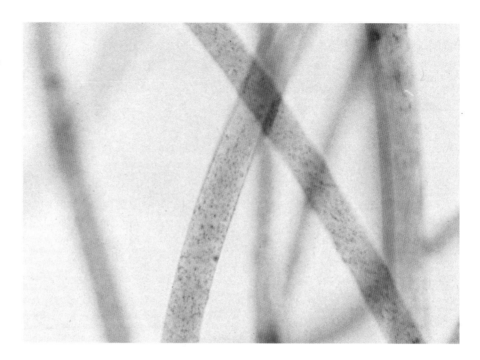

Figure I.10

*Known fibers from the
1992 Chevrolet Lumina.*

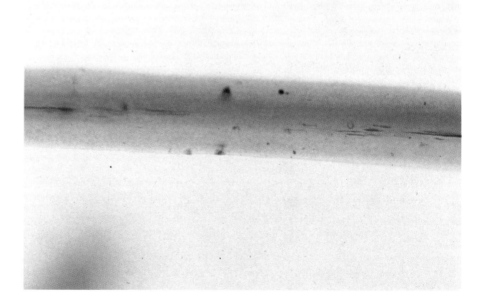

HISTORY

If we disregard Doyle and his fictional friends Holmes and Watson[2] to look at historical fact for the basis of forensic science, and in particular trace evidence, we would start in the late 1800s. Hanns Gross (1847–1915) was a professor of Criminology in the University of Prague who also spent time as a public prosecutor and judge. His classic book, *Handbuch fur Untersuchungsrichter als System dur Kriminalistik* published in 1893, stressed how important science could be to criminal investigators. The book was so successful that it was published in English as *Criminal Investigation* in 1906. As a member of the legal profession, rather than a scientist, he didn't contribute to the development of scientific methods however, in 1899 he did introduce a forensic journal entitled, *Archiv fur Kriminal – Anthropologie und Kriminalistik.*

Edmond Locard (1877–1966) made the greatest contribution in the field of scientific method development and in particular trace analysis. Locard was born in France and in 1910 he founded the anthropometric service within the Lyon Police Service. The forensic examination of trace evidence is based on a theory postulated by Locard. The theory is summarized as 'every contact leaves a trace'. Although often quoted as the Locard Exchange Principle (originally by Nickolls 1956) it is not thought to appear in any of his writing as such. Locard was also the chief editor of a forensic journal, *Revue Internationale de Criminalistique*, founded in 1929. The same year in this journal, Locard published his original paper on dust analysis in French, "L'analyse des Poussieres en Criminalistique." The phrasing, from his 1930 article "The Analysis of Dust Traces (In Three Parts)", that forms the foundation of his principle is:

> Yet, upon reflection, one is astonished that it has been necessary to wait until this late day for so simple an idea to be applied as the collecting, in the dust of garments, of the evidence of the objects rubbed against, and the contacts which a suspected person may have undergone. For the microscopic debris that cover our clothes and bodies are the mute witnesses, sure and faithful, of all our movements and of all our encounters (Locard 1930: 276).

It is interesting that, even in his day, Locard was upset at the lack of attention being paid to the examination of microscopic evidence. Locard goes on to describe the traits of dust, mud, and soil, and the examination of clothing, pockets, shoes, underwear, skin, hair, nails, ears (two and a half pages!), nostrils, weapons, and vehicles. Quite simply, Locard believed that a criminal could not visit a crime scene without leaving behind or taking away some form of trace

[2] Despite the fictional nature of the stories, the serious student of trace evidence would be well advised to read Doyle's works regarding Holmes's investigations. In particular, *A Study in Scarlet, The Five Orange Pips, The Sign of the Four, The Boscombe Valley Mystery,* and *The Resident Patient* contain intriguing, if improbable, references to trace evidence.

material. In some cases the material may be as small as a particle of dust, and, therefore, not all transfers are detectable.

Although much of the early trace work is associated with Locard, it was German-born R. A. Reiss, who, it is believed, set up the first Institute of Police Science. Reiss, who taught at the University of Lausanne, introduced a forensic photography course in the early 1900s and later his department became the Lausanne Institute of Police Science. Between 1910 and 1925, other European countries set up forensic laboratories, including France, Germany, Austria, Sweden, Finland, and Holland. In 1923 the Los Angeles Police Department set up the first forensic laboratory in the USA. August Vollmer was the main instigator and in the 1930s he was head of the Institute of Criminology and Criminalists at the University of California at Berkeley. Although the first institute of its kind in the USA, official status was only achieved in 1948 when a school of criminology was formed with Paul Kirk (1902–1970) as its head.

In 1932, with a borrowed microscope and a few other pieces of scientific equipment, the Bureau of Investigation (to be permanently renamed the Federal Bureau of Investigation in 1935) established its Technical Laboratory in Washington, DC (Figure I.11). Housed in the Justice Building at 9th Street and Pennsylvania Avenue (Figure I.12), the Laboratory was the first of its kind in the US government. The press referred to it as "a novel research laboratory where governmental criminologists (sic) will match wits with underworld cunning." The Technical Laboratory originally operated as a research facility only, with no casework being performed. With additional funding, it obtained specialized

Figure I.11
The FBI Technical Laboratory, circa 1932.

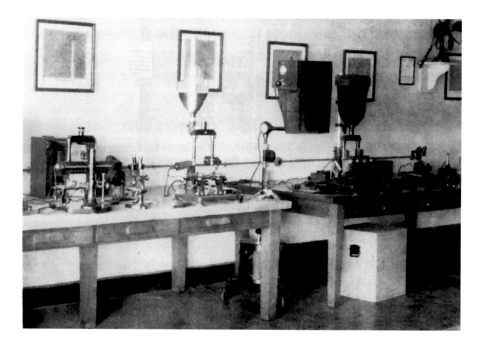

microscopes and extensive reference collections for comparisons and eventually assisted in both Federal and local investigations. The microscopic comparisons of hairs and fibers were among the first examinations authorized by the FBI Laboratory, with glass, paint, and soils soon following. During its first year of operation, the Laboratory conducted 963 examinations; currently, the Laboratory conducts well over a million examinations per year.

At about the same time as the FBI was setting up its laboratory in the USA, changes were under way in England. A number of small local authority laboratories were opening and by the mid-1930s some were moved to Home Office control. It was as a result of discussion between the Home Office and the Metropolitan Police Force in London that the Metropolitan Police Forensic Science Laboratory opened in 1935. The provincial Home Office laboratories were sited at Birmingham, Bristol, Cardiff, Harrogate, Newcastle upon Tyne, Nottingham and Preston.

Clearly, development of forensic science in the USA was behind Europe but ahead of Britain. This was to change in 1966 with the formation of the Central Research Establishment (CRE) in Aldermaston, England. The entire research program for the Home Office laboratories was housed in a building at Aldermaston and staffed by non-casework scientists. It was here that much of the early trace evidence research and development was carried out. As time passed the British laboratories merged and were re-sited until, by the mid-1970s, the Home Office laboratories were sited at Aldermaston (both casework and CRE), Birmingham, Chepstow, Chorley, Huntingdon and Wetherby.

In 1981, the FBI's Forensic Science Research and Training Center opened at Quantico, Virginia. This was the USA's answer to Britain's CRE and was the first dedicated research and development center for forensic science in the USA. Combined with the FBI's Training Academy, the Research Center provided a focus of forensic science research, teaching, and applications. Centralization continued as the theme in forensic science in the latter half of the 20th century. In 1991, the six Home Office laboratories merged to become a single agency, the Forensic Science Service. April 1996 saw the merger of the Metropolitan Police Laboratory with the Forensic Science Service (FSS). Once again, this was followed by streamlining which resulted in six laboratories being sited at Birmingham, Chepstow, Chorley, Huntingdon, London and Wetherby. Research was mainly focused in Birmingham but some was still carried out in London.

It was also in the late 1990s that it was decided that the FBI Laboratory, at that time housed in the J. Edgar Hoover Building in Washington, DC, would move to a new laboratory facility in the grounds of the FBI Academy in Quantico, Virginia (Figure I.12). The new purpose-built laboratory is currently under construction. Once again history repeats itself and as major changes happen in the USA they also happen in England. In early 2000 it was announced that the

Figure I.12

The Justice Building, Washington DC.

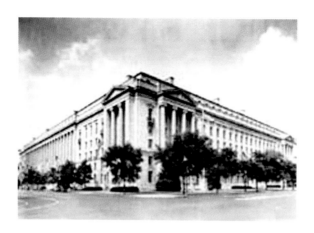

Research and Development section of the FSS would move to new premises near Birmingham International Airport, to allow for much-needed expansion and hopefully more trace research and development.

The Forensic Science Service in England, along with the FBI Laboratory in Washington, are certainly the largest forensic organizations worldwide both in staff numbers and caseload. They are also the only two organizations with large research and development sections. However, we should not forget about the contribution workers from outside these organizations have made in the past, and continue to make in many areas of trace evidence research and development.

Three of the main disciplines that provide trace evidence are fibers, paint and glass. Much of the early development work in these fields was carried out at the CRE, England. Indeed, between the mid-1970s and early 1990s many papers were published which still provide the backbone for these disciplines today. Beginning in the mid-1980s and continuing through the 1990s to the present day, our DNA colleagues have moved their discipline forward in leaps and bounds. Indeed many people thought the end of trace evidence was nigh. However, there were others who knew differently. While many of us respected the results being obtained and the resulting convictions that DNA work was achieving, we were sure it would never solve every case. With this thought in mind, a small number of experts in the trace evidence field, throughout the world, continued to publish their research, development and interpretation projects in relation to trace. In the USA it was Almirall, Bartick, DeForest, Deadman, Ryland, Suzuki, and Tungol. Europe's main workers were Allen, Evett, Grieve, Griffin, Hicks, Jackson, Lambert, Massonnet, Salter, Stocklein, and Wiggins, while in Australia and New Zealand it was Buckleton, Curran, Robertson, and Roux. There are many others, too many to list, whom, by publishing in journals, books, and proceedings have advanced the discipline of trace evidence.

Trace evidence was badly in need of a lift. It was difficult to obtain the recognition that the subject deserved when DNA was grabbing the headlines. It is true to say that the recognition that DNA was getting was justifiably deserved. However, in late 1993 and early 1994, two trace workers in Europe and a research scientist in the USA decided it was time to take action.

Ken Wiggins from the Metropolitan Police Forensic Science Laboratory (now the London Laboratory of the FSS) and Mike Grieve from the US Army Crime Laboratory in Frankfurt, Germany (now working at the Forensic Science Institute of the Budeskriminalamt, Wiesbaden, Germany) decided, with the co-operation of their respective organizations, to establish the European Fibres Group. The first meeting of the group was held in The Hague, The Netherlands in November 1993. Twenty-one scientists from 17 laboratories in 12 European countries attended the meeting. The current membership is approaching 80 scientists from 49 laboratories in 23 European countries. In addition, representatives from Australia, Canada, Israel, and the USA regularly attend its meetings.

At the first meeting four aims were agreed upon. The first was to meet regularly and informally with the minimum of bureaucracy, allowing as many different laboratories as possible to be represented from across Europe. The only stipulation is that the participants should be actively concerned with fiber examination. The group agreed to meet on a yearly basis: as the group performs collaborative trials on a yearly basis it is essential to discuss the results and implications as soon as possible; collaborative research results need to be disseminated to the group quickly; it is very important that the group is kept up to date with current developments.

The second aim was to promote the exchange of knowledge, experiences and information between specialists concerning all aspects of the examination of textiles, especially methods of retrieval, comparison, and identification.

Standardization – the third aim – is critical to trace evidence despite differing legal systems and their requirements, and varying availability of equipment within different laboratories. The group is confident that it will be able to work towards standardization of techniques and instrumental methods and is at present working on a project which will result in the production of a Manual of Best Practice for Forensic Fibre Examination.

The fourth aim is collaborative research, which is a very valuable cost- and time-saver that tends to counteract the increasing shortage of manpower and resources.

The European Fibres Group now falls under the European Network of Forensic Science Institute's (ENFSI) umbrella, as do most of the European

Working Groups. The Australian guests are representing the Criminalistic Scientific Advisory Group, a group nominated by the Senior Managers of Australia and New Zealand Forensic Laboratories (SMANZFL), whereas the Americans represent the Scientific Working Group for Materials (SWGMAT). In addition, relations are developing between the EFG and South Africa and Japan.

SWGMAT was formed under the name of the Technical Working Group for Fibers in 1994 by Edward Bartick of the FBI. A similar group for paint debuted soon after and FBI management recognized the need to have all of the trace disciplines in one Group. Thus, TWGFIBE became TWGMAT, for materials, and Max M. Houck of the FBI Laboratory's Trace Evidence Unit became the chairman in 1996. TWGMAT became SWGMAT in 1999 to reflect the more scientific nature of its goals. It is made up of bench-level scientists who are dedicated to the preservation and improvement of trace evidence collection, analysis, and testimony. It is currently divided into Fibers, Paint, Glass, Tape, and Hair sub-groups.

The work undertaken by SWGMAT falls into three categories: guidelines, analytical projects and technical papers. The projects include round-robin style research and surveys while the technical papers convey and document matters of scientific, analytical, or industrial information. The group has been working toward the production of guidelines for each of the disciplines; the first document "Forensic Fiber Examination Guidelines" was published in January 1998 and is currently available in *Forensic Science Communications*, an on-line FBI journal at www.fbi.gov. American fiber examiners wrote the document with assistance from colleagues in Canada, England, and Germany. Indeed it is this document on which colleagues in Europe are basing their Manual of Best Practice for Forensic Fibre Examination.

Currently SWGMAT's membership stands at 84 people representing 46 laboratories in 28 states and 8 countries. Invited guests attend meetings from the European Fibre and Paint groups, the Australian Scientific Advisory groups, Canada, South Africa, and Japan.

In 1995, Wilfreid Stocklein of the Forensic Science Institute of the Bundeskriminalamt in Wiesbaden, Germany established the European Paint Group. The membership is 33 laboratories in 22 European and 3 non-European countries. The aims of the group were defined as:

■ Establishment of collections and databases (including education and training in their use) concerning paint, for the benefit of all paint examiners.

■ Development of guidelines for paint examination casework-related communication and exchange of scientific news to form the basis of informal co-operation with a minimum of bureaucracy.

■ Introduction of a collaborative proficiency testing program.

■ Co-ordination of research projects.

These aims are very much in line with those of SWGMAT and the EFG. In 1999 a glass section was attached to the EPG.

The formation of SWGMAT and its European counterparts has gone a long way to lifting the profile of trace evidence over the last seven years. These groups are actually improving this subject area and, by working closely together, have had a major impact on improving the knowledge of trace evidence examiners worldwide.

THE IMPORTANCE OF TRANSFER EVIDENCE

As previously stated, the types of trace evidence that may be encountered by the forensic scientist are vast:

> Wherever he steps, whatever he touches, whatever he leaves, even unconsciously, will serve as silent witness against him. Not just his fingerprints or his footprints, but his hair, the fibers from his clothes, the glass he breaks, the tool marks he leaves, the paint he scratches, the blood or semen he deposits or collects – all of these bear mute witness against him. This is evidence that does not forget. It is not confused by the excitement of the moment. It is not absent because human witnesses are. It is factual evidence. Physical evidence cannot be wrong; it cannot perjure itself, it cannot be wholly absent – only its interpretation can err. Only human failure to find it, study and understand it, can diminish its value. (Harris v United States, 331US145, 1947)

This statement was made over fifty years ago but its content still holds true today. The scientist does not have the time to search for the transfer of all trace evidence in every case. He has to be selective and prioritize.

Before benchwork begins, the scientist generally carries out an assessment of the information available and the items provided for examination in relation to the work request. He may wish to consider to what extent the proposition put forward by the police can be tested and should consider an alternative hypothesis put forward by the defense. If this course of action is followed he should consider what he would expect to find if either proposition were correct. At this time the likely evidential value of the anticipated findings should be considered, and, depending on the type of trace material, the considerations may differ. Irrespective of these considerations, certain information will always be required, if available, on:

- what is the defense and/or what is the suspect saying,
- what is suspected or known to have happened, before, during, and after the incident,
- the persons involved, and their relationships (spouses, strangers, etc.),

- the sequence and timings of events,
- the nature of the surfaces/textiles that may have come into contact,
- the persons responsible for and the sequence and timing of events in the recovery of items submitted for examination.

Contamination has always been an issue for all trace evidence examiners in forensic science. It is important that everyone in the forensic process is aware of contamination and takes appropriate action to minimize the risk. Casework material is vulnerable from the moment a crime is committed, so the risk of contamination can become an issue long before exhibits arrive at the forensic science laboratory.

There is enormous pressure on the first officer attending a scene and also those responsible for the subsequent management of the scene to avoid contamination. Once the interactions between the victim(s), the suspect(s), and the crime scene have ceased, any further contact between these items constitutes contamination. It is vital that anyone who has attended the scene or been involved with the packaging of control samples has no contact with the suspect or their clothing. Situations should be avoided where the same officer takes possession of clothing from a suspect and victim in the same case. In addition multiple suspects, the victim, and their clothing must be kept apart at all times and should not be allowed to come into contact with the same objects or people, for example, police car, interview room, custody rooms, or emergency rooms, among others. Finally, the same officer should not search a property and then deal with persons or objects linked to the property. It goes without saying, or at least it should, that all exhibits should be packaged separately and sealed as soon as they are taken. Once these general personnel issues have been addressed there are anti-contamination precautions that should be taken both at the scene and in the laboratory.

Appropriate anti-contamination precautions should be taken at the scene to minimize any chance of accidental contamination of items that may subsequently be required for laboratory examination. Consideration of what anti-contamination precaution to take should be based on all the evidence types that may be potentially available. Generally the wearing of protective clothing such as disposable jumpsuits, gloves and facemasks is desirable. In addition all equipment, sampling materials, and storage and transportation containers should be new, preferably disposable, or cleaned thoroughly before and after each use. It is particularly important that adhesive tape used for taping evidence should be kept in its container or other packaging whenever it is not in use.

All items submitted to the laboratory for trace evidence examination should first be examined for the integrity of their packaging. Any deficiency in the packaging which may compromise the value of a laboratory examination may be grounds for refusal to carry out the laboratory examination. Scientists and technicians should wear protective clothing to minimize the risk of trace evidence transfer from the examiner to the items being examined and secondary transfer between items via the examiner. Ideally, different personnel or rooms should be employed to process items from a victim and from a suspect. When this is not possible, there must be a clear time interval and evidence of decontamination between searches. Items should preferably be searched in purpose-designed rooms with restricted access and air filtration. Benches used for searching should be rigorously cleaned prior to any examination and the rooms should be cleaned regularly. Different rooms should be used to search items from different scenes or people and these rooms should be physically separate (for example, doors or permanent partitions) from each other. Dedicated laboratory coats, which should be labeled, and equipment should be provided for use within each search room. Tape dispensers, if used, should be enclosed to prevent contamination by stray airborne fibers.

QUANTITY AND TYPE OF TRANSFERRED TRACE EVIDENCE MATERIAL

In order to be able to assess the potential significance of any findings, it is important to have information about the type and quantity of trace material that may have been present at the time of the offense. Was the suspect wearing a fluffy acrylic sweater that would shed fibers readily or was he wearing a nylon jacket that would normally shed very few fibers? Alternatively, if a murder resulted after a fight began in a lumberyard would we expect the suspect's clothing to be covered in wood fragments and sawdust? The quantity would depend on the contact made. If the suspect and victim "rolled around" on the ground then their clothing is likely to be contaminated with sawdust. However, if the suspect remained on his feet it is less likely that there will be large quantities of sawdust on his clothing.

LOCATING AND RECOVERY OF TRACE MATERIALS

The more trace material transferred at the time of the offence should make the location and recovery that much easier. However, one of the most important aspects when trying to locate trace material is its size. The vast range of samples covered by the words "trace material" has already been mentioned but the common denominator is size. A tuft of hair, a large paint flake or a pill of fibers can all be seen by eye, hence making location and recovery easy. However, finding evidence like this is rare for the reasons given in the section below on persistence. It is far more likely that the trace material will be microscopic in size and hence location and recovery is more difficult.

Trace material may be recovered (generally within the confines of the laboratory) by picking off with forceps, taping, combing, brushing, vacuuming, shaking, or scraping. Each evidence type can be collected using one or more of the techniques listed above. Every laboratory or scientist will no doubt have their own ideas as to the best method for each specific evidence type. It may be advisable or desirable to recover some trace evidence at the scene. If this is the case then taping, possibly using a 1:1 taping method, or picking off with forceps would be the commonest techniques employed.

In any case or scenario time also becomes important in transfer of trace material. How long were the items of interest in contact? Generally, longer contact would mean a greater chance of material being transferred. Another consideration is the length of time since the crime occurred. A body that has been exposed for several days may have a different retention of trace materials than one that has been inside for the same amount of time (Spencer 1994: 894).

PERSISTENCE OF TRACE MATERIAL

There are many issues that affect the persistence of trace material.

- The size and texture of the material being transferred; that is, is the material large or small, is it rough or smooth?
- The surface on which it is being retained; once again is it rough or smooth?
- Can brushing, washing, or vacuuming easily remove the transferred material? Has the suspect tried to remove it?
- The length of time interval between offense and recovery of retained material.
- The degree of activity by the suspect/victim if the retaining material is clothing.

Using the lumberyard fight and subsequent murder discussed above as a scenario, the persistence issues can be put into perspective.

Large wood fragments are less likely to be retained on clothing but sawdust may well be found. If the retentive surface is smooth, sawdust may not adhere but it may be found in pockets. If no attempt has been made by the suspect to clean his clothes then the chances of finding trace evidence is increased. If the suspect rolled in the sawdust during the fight then more sawdust is likely to have been transferred to him. The question of what the suspect did after the offense and before the time of his arrest also become relevant. If he sat down at the scene and waited to be arrested then very little evidence would be lost. However, if he ran from the scene and when he got home, brushed the outside of his clothing and the inside of his pockets carefully, before washing it, then the volume of trace material left is likely to be less.

EVALUATION AND INTERPRETATION OF TRACE MATERIAL

If we spend the time and effort searching for trace material and we find it, how are we going to evaluate/interpret what it means? Will it add anything to the case either for the defense or prosecution? Searching for white cotton is a waste of time as it is prevalent in the general fiber population worldwide. However, searching for, and finding, a 12-layer paint fragment on a suspect which is identical in all tested characteristics to a sample from the point of entry is likely to provide very good evidence. This is particularly true if the suspect denies even being in the vicinity of the scene.

The same type of information is required for the evaluation and interpretation of the evidence found during the examination of a case as is required for the case assessment undertaken before commencing any examination. Indeed, if the case assessment has been carried out thoroughly the evaluation and interpretation of the case findings should be straightforward.

In order to evaluate and interpret the case findings, a number of points need to be considered:

- any case-related background information together with any hypotheses formulated during case assessment,
- contamination risks,
- the transfer and retentive properties of material(s) involved,
- the amount and type(s) of trace material found,
- the degree of specificity/certainty that can be attached to the identification of the trace material,
- the commonness of the material,
- the level of discrimination achieved when the material is compared, and
- whether a one-way or two-way transfer of material(s) is involved.

The quality of any evaluation of evidential significance will depend on the quality of the information on which it is based. Unfortunately, there will rarely be any situation where all the information requirements are met, and the quality of what information is available may be very varied. There will always be an element of subjectivity in how this is used and what weight should be attached to the different aspects. This is where the judgment and expertise of the expert witness comes in.

In addition to information relating directly to the case itself, there are other sources of information available to assist in the interpretation of trace evidence. These include: reference collections, frequency databases, commercial data, published forensic and other literature.

Finally, how can the evidential significance of trace evidence be evaluated? A method of assessing the influence of the various factors is to use the Bayesian approach. This is where the evidence is considered under two competing hypotheses, one based on the prosecution allegation and the other on a defense position, i.e. "what are the chances of finding the trace evidence if the suspect is the person who sat in the car seat?" against "what is the chance of finding the trace evidence if the suspect is not the person who sat in the car seat?". In very simple terms, by applying best estimates to each of the relevant factors considered, an assessment can be made for the probability of the evidence under each hypothesis and from this the Likelihood Ratio (LR) can be approximated. Depending on the magnitude of the LR, one or other of the propositions is favored. Once in court the LR can be expressed in terms of a standard verbal scale of strength of evidence indicating the extent to which the findings support one or other of the propositions.

It is important to stress that for most trace evidence the use of a Bayesian approach cannot offer precise numerical assessment of probabilities involved. Although this may be the ultimate and desirable situation, the merits of the Bayesian approach probably lie elsewhere. The Bayesian framework provides the basic principles – the building blocks, the inferential engine – for interpreting evidence. The principles are:

- Interpretation of scientific evidence is carried out within a framework of circumstances. The interpretation depends on the structure and content of the framework.
- Interpretation is only meaningful when two or more competing propositions are considered.
- The role of the forensic scientist is to consider the probability of the evidence given the propositions that are considered.

In trace evidence, all assessments made in the third point above will be based on various sources of data; some may involve statistical figures and others may stem from manufacturers' information or experience. The final assessment will rarely be expressed through a number (giving an illusory precision) but by subjective assessment, giving a level of confidence that can be sustained by overall data.

A potential danger with a likelihood ratio is that the court and the jury may give more evidentiary weight to an apparently "quantitative" method that may not have a more factual basis than the examiner's professional opinion. The public expects a mathematical approach from a scientist (Houck 1999) and numbers can heavily influence juries. Although this may be true for some evidence types it would be rare to find any report relating to trace evidence, written adopting a Bayesian approach, which concludes with a numerical estimate of the likelihood ratio. The data which is currently available to trace evidence examiners would be insufficient to achieve such precision. The use of and research in Bayes' Theorem with its perceived numerical approach has generated numerous publications but most adherents are European with little interest or application in the United States. The current view in the USA is that because the data are estimated and may be based on "vague" probabilities (Grieve 1994), Bayes Theorem does not solve the persistent problematic situation in the United States' courts: the very strong adversarial system. Experts may differ in their opinions about evidentiary significance because of the various background information, their professional experiences, and the baseline date they are using. This, however, is not a consequence of the Bayesian approach; it is a consequence of the subjective nature of data interpretation within a scientific method. Certainly, the interest in the Bayesean approach has generated useful discussion of evidential interpretation and value. As previously stated, this method of assessment is used more readily in Europe, in particular the UK, rather than in the USA. Only time will tell if it becomes accepted as a practice worldwide.

This introduction shows, we hope, that trace evidence is not standing still and that experts in the field worldwide are still trying to improve and develop this particular discipline. The reader should also now be aware of the amount and type of thought and reasoning that goes into every case even prior to starting any examination. It hopefully dispels the myth that trace evidence is dead. With the right training and given the time to find it, trace evidence can be a very powerful weapon in the fight against crime.

REFERENCES

Grieve, M.C. (1994) "Fibers and forensic science – new ideas, developments and techniques", *For. Sci. Int.*, 6, 60.

Houck, M.M. "Statistics and trace evidence: the tyranny of numbers," *Forensic Science Communications* [On-line] V1, N3. Available at www.fbi.gov.

Kirk, P.L. (1953) *Crime Investigation*. New York: John Wiley & Sons.

Locard, E. (1929) "L'analyse des Poussieres en Criminalistique," *Revue Internationale de Criminalistique*, nos. 4–5, 176–249.

Locard, E. (1930) *Am. J. Police Sci.*, 6, 276–298.

Nickolls, L.C. (1956) *The Scientific Investigation of Crime*. London: Butterworth & Co. Ltd.

Spencer, R. (1994) *J. For. Sci.*, 39, 894.

CHAPTER 1

FABRIC PROCESSING AND "NUBS"[1]

Douglas W. Deedrick

INTRODUCTION

Violent physical contact often results in the transfer of minute traces of evidence that may be overlooked by the crime scene examiner and the forensic scientist. The experience levels of the collector and forensic examiner help drive the direction and scope of evidentiary searches and analyses. Past successes in fingerprint and DNA identifications may place emphasis on a select few items of physical evidence and other critical evidence may be overlooked or discounted. A complete understanding of the mechanisms of evidence transfer during the commission of a violent crime can add a considerable number of additional "pieces of the puzzle." The recovery, identification and comparison of minute traces of hair, fiber, soil, glass, feathers, paint chips, etc. can often provide invaluable insight into the nature of the contact and the identity of the perpetrator.

The transfer of hairs and fibers and their discovery as trace evidence can be critical in associating a suspect to a victim or to a crime scene. Effective use of hair and fiber evidence, however, requires an understanding of its dynamic nature. Knowing how hairs and fibers can be transferred and which factors affect the significance of a hair or fiber match are important concerns of crime scene technicians, laboratory examiners, investigators, and prosecutors.

Whenever a fiber found on the clothing of a victim matches the known fibers of a suspect's clothing, it can be a significant event. Matching dyed synthetic fibers or dyed natural fibers can be very meaningful, whereas the matching of common fibers such as white cotton or blue denim cotton would be less significant. In some situations, however, the presence of white cotton or blue denim cotton may still have some meaning in resolving the truth of an issue. The discovery of cross-transfers and multiple fiber transfers between the suspect's clothing and the victim's clothing dramatically increases the likelihood that these two individuals had physical contact.

When a fiber examiner matches a questioned fiber to a known item of clothing, there are only two possible explanations: the fiber actually originated from the item of clothing, or the fiber did not originate from the item of

[1] Portions of this chapter were originally published in "Hairs, Fibers, Crime, and Evidence," *Forensic Science Communications* [On-line] V2, N3, available at www.fbi.gov.

clothing. In order to say that the fiber originated from the item of clothing, the clothing either had to be the only fabric of its type ever produced or still remaining on earth, or the transfer of fibers was directly observed. Since neither of these situations is likely to occur or be known, fiber examiners will conclude that the fibers could have originated from the clothing or that the fibers are consistent with originating from the clothing. The only way to say that a fiber did not originate from a particular item of clothing is to know the actual history of the garment or to have actually observed the fiber transfer from another garment.

It is argued that the large volume of fabric produced reduces the significance of any fiber association discovered in a criminal case. It can never be stated with certainty that a fiber originated from a particular garment because other garments were likely produced using the same fiber type and color. The inability to positively associate a fiber with a particular garment to the exclusion of all other garments, however, does not mean that the fiber association is without value.

When one considers the volume of fabric produced in the world each year, the number of garments of a particular color and fiber type is extremely small. The likelihood of two or more manufacturers duplicating all aspects of the fabric type and color exactly is extremely remote. The large number of dye types and colors that exist in the world, coupled with the unlimited number of possible dye combinations, makes any fiber association by color significant. One must also consider the lifespan of a particular fabric: only so much of a given fabric of a particular color and fiber type is produced, and it will eventually end up being destroyed or dumped in a landfill.

More than 100 billion pounds of fiber were produced in 1998. Approximately 40 billion pounds of cotton were used to produce textile products during 1998 (*Fiber Organon* 1999), and although a great many of these fibers were used in the production of clothing, a large amount of cotton fiber was also used for other purposes, such as stuffing and padding material (batting), cotton swabs, and cotton balls. Much of the cotton used in clothing ends up undyed, as in white shirts, underwear, socks, and bed sheets, but often cotton is dyed many different shades of blue, red, green, and yellow. Much of the cotton fabric produced is also print-dyed, which imparts different color characteristics to the surface of the cotton fibers, and some cotton fabrics are dyed in such a way as to vary the color along the length of the fiber. The cotton fibers in fabrics can remain in a rough state or can be processed in different ways, such as by mercerization.

Another important consideration is coincidence. When fibers that match the clothing fibers of the suspect are found on the clothing of a victim, two conclusions may be drawn: the fibers originated from the suspect, or the fibers originated from another fabric source that not only was composed of fibers of the exact type and color, but was also in a position to contribute those fibers through primary or secondary contact. The likelihood of encountering identical fibers from the environment of a homicide victim (i.e. from his or her residence or friends) is extremely remote.

The initial stages of a crime scene investigation are critical because valuable physical evidence can be lost, destroyed or altered by individuals not directly responsible for documenting, recording and recovering the evidence. The position of the body, the specific location of individual items of evidence and the immediate area around the body can provide invaluable clues toward the solution of the crime. Control of the scene is especially important when considering the presence or absence of trace materials like hairs and fibers. These types of materials can easily be transferred to and from individuals having uncontrolled contact with the body and scene.

The manner in which a crime scene is searched is determined by the type of crime, the location of the scene, details concerning events of the crime, the time of day, the number of people available for the search, and available equipment. Inasmuch as hair and fiber evidence can play a role in most cases involving violent crime, serious consideration should be given to collecting it properly. Once the crime has been committed, little time remains before hair and fiber evidence will be lost or contaminated. The importance of securing the crime scene cannot be overstated.

When physical contact occurs between two individuals, objects, or individuals and objects, there is a likelihood of transfer of hair and fiber evidence. This likelihood is dependent on the nature of the contact, the duration of the contact, and the nature of the contacting surfaces. The direct transfer of hairs from the head of an individual to the clothing of another individual is called a primary transfer. When hairs have already been shed and are transferred to an individual, it is called secondary transfer. Fibers are transferred in a similar manner. When fibers are transferred from the fabric of an individual's clothing to the clothing of another individual, it is called a primary transfer. As these same fibers are transferred to other objects during subsequent contacts, secondary transfers are occurring.

It is important for crime scene investigators to understand the mechanisms of primary and secondary transfer. As trace evidence can be transferred during the commission of a crime, it can also be transferred during the search process. Investigators can not only pick up hairs and fibers inadvertently, they can be inadvertently deposited at the crime scene. The following are considerations at the crime scene:

- Elimination hair and/or fiber samples may need to be obtained from personnel conducting the search.
- Prioritize the order of evidence collection. Collect large items first and then proceed to the trace evidence. *Use caution when walking through the crime scene.*
- Taping, or tweezing, take blood samples, remove bullets, dust for fingerprints, and so on.
- Processing the crime scene for fingerprints prior to trace evidence collection is not recommended because it can:
  - inadvertently transfer trace evidence onto the clothing of the technicians,
  - move trace evidence, and/or
  - contaminate trace evidence with dusting powder.

The following are suggestions for collecting evidence from crime scenes such as houses, apartments, and vehicles:

- Photograph all evidence prior to removing it.
- Remove larger items or debris from carpeting or walk areas prior to other examinations. Consider wearing disposable booties.
- Collect large items, such as clothing, and place them in separate paper bags. Keep an accurate evidence log. One person should collect and bag the items while another person labels the bags and records the items in the log.
- Do not place all clothing items from a suspect in one paper bag, or all items from a victim in another bag. Bag each item separately.
- Never put suspect items and victim items in contact with one another. The person collecting the suspect's items should not be the same person that collects the victim's items. If this must occur, personnel must change their clothing and collect the evidence at a different time to avoid contamination.
- Bedding should be carefully handled to avoid loss of hairs and fibers. Each item should be placed in a separate bag.
- Floor surfaces should be vacuumed for possible trace evidence. Some crime scene investigators use tape to secure trace evidence; however, tape is generally difficult to work with at the scene and in the laboratory. Smaller surfaces such as chairs and car seats can be taped or vacuumed.
- Ensure that carpet, pet hair, and other standards that might have transferred to a suspect or victim are collected.
- Always process for fingerprints after collecting trace evidence.
- Collect all possible known fiber samples from a vehicle. These may be obtained from the carpet, door panels, headliner, seats, floor mats, and trunk.
- *Hats:* Package all hats in separate paper bags. Use care when collecting baseball-style caps with adjustable plastic headbands – the bands are an excellent source for fingerprints.

- *Shoes:* Shoes are an excellent source of fiber evidence, bloodstains, and shoe print comparisons. Shoes worn by a suspect can deposit fibers from a vehicle he or she exited at a crime scene and can also pick up fibers from the scene and then deposit them in another location.

- *Socks:* Socks worn by a homicide victim can provide invaluable fiber and hair evidence. Many times the victim is transported by vehicle. Contact with the interior surfaces of a vehicle can cause hairs and fibers to collect on the socks. It may be necessary to obtain elimination samples of the carpeting of the victim's car or residence to avoid the possibility of a coincidental match.

- *Fingernails:* Use care when scraping or clipping the fingernails of a victim or suspect. DNA on the hands or tools of the medical personnel can contaminate the material and influence the DNA results.

- *Hairs in the hands of the victim:* Hairs found in the hands of the victim usually belong to the victim. Rarely are the hairs similar to the suspect's known hairs; nevertheless, these must be collected and submitted for analysis.

- *Pubic and head hair combings:* Pubic and head hair combings should always be taken in violent crimes. Foreign hairs as well as fibers can be recovered from these samples. If a hat is recovered at the crime scene and a suspect is identified soon, it may be possible to find fibers similar to those in the hat in the suspect's hair.

- *Known hair samples:* Thorough random samples should be taken from the head and pubic regions of a suspect(s) and victim(s). Twenty-five full-length hairs, pulled and combed from different areas of the head and pubic regions, are generally considered an adequate representation of an individual's hair characteristics.

- *Weapons:* Weapons recovered at a crime scene should always be searched for trace evidence before processing for fingerprints.

- *Doors and windows:* Doors and windows should be searched for trace evidence if they are possible points of entry or exit.

Once the evidence has been collected, there are several recommendations or considerations when packaging it for transmittal to the laboratory. Clothing items must be packaged in separate sealed paper bags – not plastic. To avoid contamination, clothing items from the suspect should never be handled in the same area in which items from the victim are handled. All damp or blood-soaked items must be air-dried in a room away from air movement and traffic. Drying paper placed under damp clothing items should be submitted separately.

Submit individual hairs and fibers in clean paper or in an envelope with sealed corners. The primary paper or envelope should be placed inside a secondary sealed envelope with all corners taped. Many times individual hairs identified on items of clothing are not removed or secured. These hairs may move or be lost, so it is recommended that they be removed and placed in an envelope (first noting where they were removed from).

On August 22, 1995, the body of eight-year-old Sandra Price[2] was discovered in a small wooded area. Sandra had been brutally assaulted and strangled just blocks from her home. She had been riding her bicycle in a church parking lot in her neighborhood and concerns for her safety arose when she failed to return at the appointed time. A search of the wooded area near the church disclosed the body and the local police were notified. The scene now came under the control of local law enforcement and a team of crime scene investigators began a detailed search of the immediate area.

The bicycle Sandra had been riding had been tossed to one side and her body had been partially hidden by overhanging branches. The bicycle was collected in the hopes that fingerprints on the frame might reveal the identity of the murderer. Her body was carefully placed in a clean sheet and then a body bag; she was transported to the coroner's office for a more detailed examination. At the coroner's office, debris was recovered from her fingernails, abdomen and hands. Vaginal swabs and rectal swabs from a standard sex crimes kit were used to recover additional items of physical evidence. Her swimsuit top, bottom, shorts, and sandals were carefully packaged in individual brown paper bags. The sheet used to transport the victim was also packaged in a brown paper bag. Known samples of blood and hair were collected.

THE ANALYSIS

The evidence recovered from the victim was delivered to a regional forensic laboratory where analyses identified DNA on her body and fingerprints on the bicycle she had been riding. Hair evidence and fiber evidence was also recovered from the victim's clothing but the initial findings were limited. The examination of the vaginal and rectal swabs and the victim's swimsuit and shorts failed to reveal the presence of semen. Fingerprint evidence from the bicycle also offered no leads. Forensic comparisons of crime scene evidence with samples obtained from an early suspect in the case failed to reveal an association. From the outset, it appeared that little would be found that could identify the murderer.

Intensive investigation by detectives assigned to the case identified an individual who might have been responsible for the death of Sandra Price. Everett Bell, a local resident, was questioned regarding the homicide; work shirts, a pair of pants, and a cap that had been provided to him by his employer, a local Hardees restaurant, were turned over to the police (Figures 1.1 and 1.2). Interviews of the Hardees manager and co-workers revealed that on the day of the murder, Bell had been sent home early from work for horseplay. An individual matching Bell's description had been seen riding his bicycle in the victim's neighborhood around the time of the homicide. The items seized from Bell

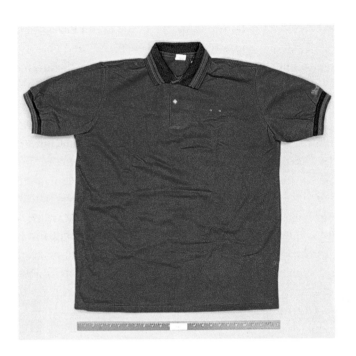

Figure 1.1
Clothes from suspect.

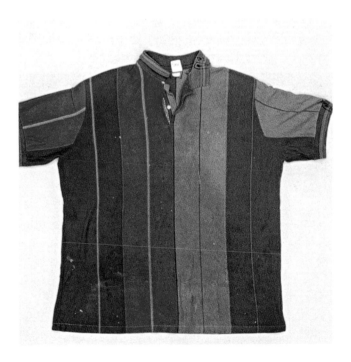

Figure 1.2
Clothes from suspect.

and the items collected from the victim at autopsy were forwarded to the FBI Laboratory for analysis.

The evidence submitted to the FBI Laboratory included numerous items recovered from the victim's body, her clothing and a known head hair sample. Two work shirts, a pair of pants, and a cap from the suspect also were submitted. Two additional work shirts from the Hardees restaurant and a shirt from Angelica Uniform Group, the supplier of the uniforms for Hardees, were also received. The individual containers of debris from the victim and the swabs from the rape kit were carefully examined using a stereo-binocular microscope. Hair and fiber evidence was mounted on glass microscope slides for identification and comparison. The victim's swimsuit top and bottoms, her sandals and her shorts were thoroughly examined in an evidence processing room. Trace evidence, mostly hairs and fibers, recovered from these items was preserved in pillboxes and later would be mounted on separate glass microscope slides. Using the suspect's work clothing as known fiber standards, the questioned fibers recovered from the victim's body and clothing were compared using a comparison microscope to determine whether or not physical contact could have occurred between the suspect and the victim (Figure 1.3). The questioned and known fibers were further compared using polarized light, fluorescence and microspectrophotometry.

The fingernail clippings and swabs from the victim revealed blue cotton fibers matching the blue cotton fibers from one of the suspect's shirts (Figures 1.4 and 1.5). Also in the fingernail clippings, on a swab from the victim's knee,

Figure 1.3

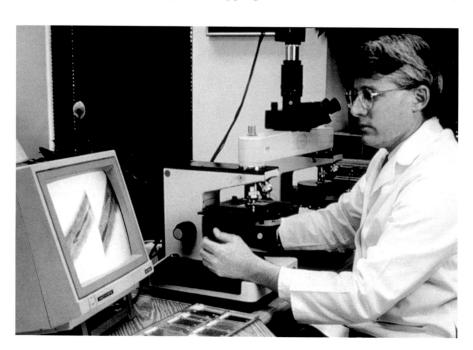

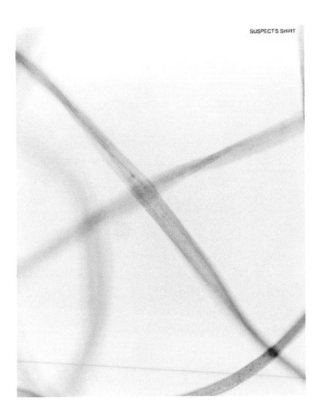

Figure 1.4
Blue cotton from suspect's shirt.

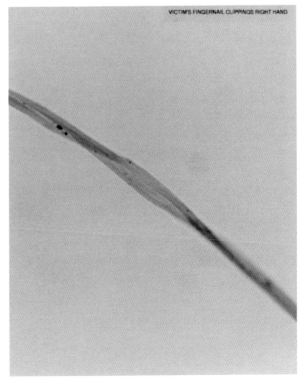

Figure 1.5
Blue cotton found in victim's fingernail clippings.

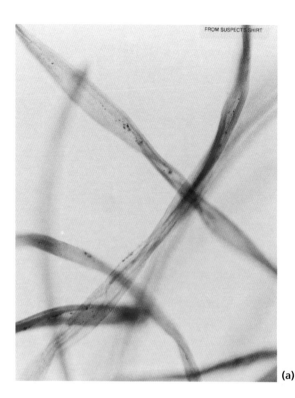
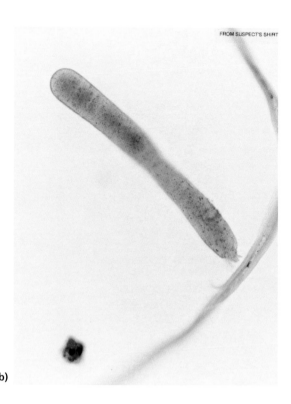

(a)   (b)

Figure 1.6

(a) Blue-green cotton fibers from suspect's shirt. (b) Blue ployester from suspect's shirt.

Figure 1.7 (opposite, above)

(a) Blue-green cotton fibers found on victim's swimsuit top. (b) Blue polyester found on victim's left knee.

Figure 1.8 (opposite, below)

(a, b) Blue polyester found on victim's swimsuit top.

and on the swimsuit were found blue-green cotton fibers (Figures 1.6a, 1.6b, 1.7a and 1.7b), blue polyester fibers (Figures 1.8a, 1.8b, 1.9a and 1.9b), and blue-green polyester fibers matching the same shirt from the suspect (Figures 1.10 and 1.11). A dark blue-gray polyester fiber matching the suspect's pant fibers was found on the rectal swab (Figures 1.12 and 1.13). Of particular interest were two different colors of melted polyester "nubs" found on the victim's items that matched polyester nubs found on the surface of the suspect's shirt.

Negroid limb hairs and hair fragments were also found on the victim's items. Hairs from the legs and arms constitute limb hairs. These hairs are shorter in length, arc-like in shape, and often abraded or tapered at the tips. The pigment in limb hair is generally granular in appearance, and the medulla is trace to discontinuous.

While limb hairs are not routinely compared in a forensic laboratory, they can differ in appearance between individuals. These differences, however, are not considered sufficient to allow limb hairs to be of value for meaningful comparison purposes. The presence of leg or arm hairs on certain items of evidence may help to corroborate other investigative information.

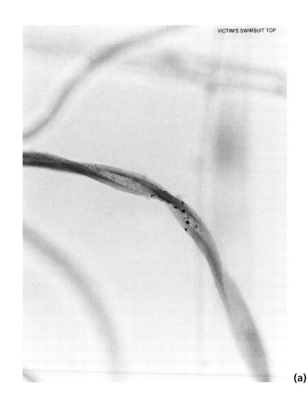

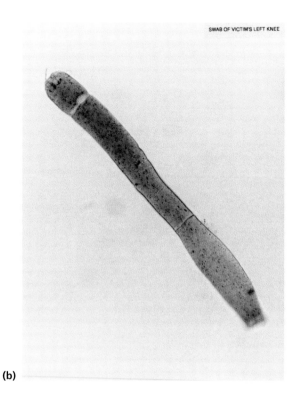

(a)   (b)

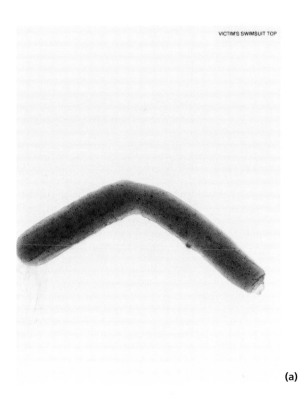

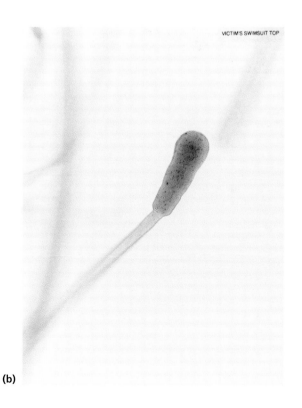

(a)   (b)

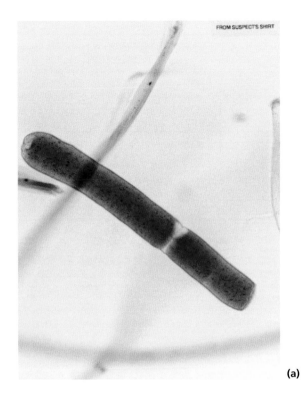

(a)   (b)

Figure 1.9
(a, b) Blue polyester from
suspect's shirt.

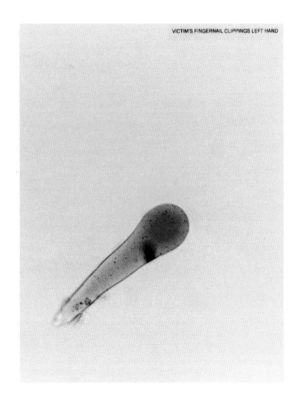

Figure 1.10
Blue-green polyester found
in victim's fingernail
clippings.

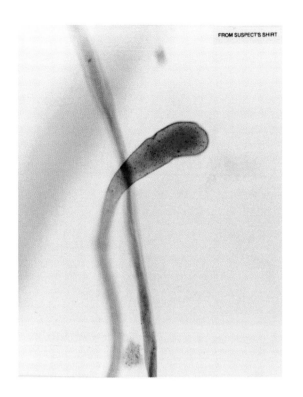

Figure 1.11
Blue-green polyester from suspect's shirt.

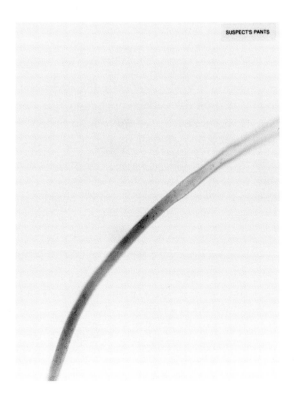

Figure 1.12
Dark blue-gray polyester fiber from suspect's pants.

Figure 1.13

Dark blue-gray polyester fiber from victim's rectal swab.

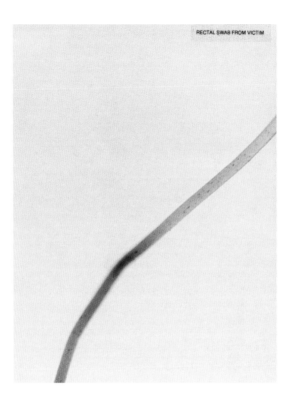

RECTAL SWAB FROM VICTIM

INTERPRETATION

As stated previously, violent physical contact often results in the transfer of trace evidence. The finding of multiple fiber matches in this case was extremely significant in linking Everett Bell to the murder of Sandra Price. While the presence of Negroid hairs and hair fragments does not specifically link Bell, their presence is consistent with the nature of the physical contact.

A fiber is the smallest unit of a textile material that has a length many times greater than its diameter. Fibers can occur naturally as plant and animal fibers, but they can also be man-made. A fiber can be spun with other fibers to form a yarn that can be woven or knitted to form a fabric. The type and length of fiber used, the type of spinning method, and the type of fabric construction all affect the transfer of fibers and the significance of fiber associations. This becomes very important when there is a possibility of fiber transfer between a suspect and a victim during the commission of a crime.

As discussed previously, fibers are considered a form of trace evidence that can be transferred from the clothing of a suspect to the clothing of a victim during the commission of a crime. Fibers can also transfer from a fabric source such as a carpet, bed, or furniture at a crime scene. These transfers can either be direct (primary) or indirect (secondary). A primary transfer occurs when a fiber is transferred from a fabric directly onto a victim's clothing, whereas a secondary transfer occurs when already transferred fibers on the clothing of a suspect transfer to the clothing of a victim. An understanding of the mechanics of primary and secondary transfer is important when reconstructing the events of a crime.

When two people come in contact or when contact occurs with an item from the crime scene, the possibility exists that a fiber transfer will take place. This does not mean that a fiber transfer will always take place. Certain types of fabric do not shed well (donor garments), and some fabrics do not hold fibers well (recipient garments). The construction and fiber composition of the fabric, the duration and force of contact, and the condition of the garment with regard to damage are important considerations.

An important consideration is the length of time between the actual physical contact and the collection of clothing items from the suspect or victim. If the victim is immobile, very little fiber loss will take place, whereas the suspect's clothing will lose transferred fibers quickly. The likelihood of finding transferred fibers on the clothing of the suspect a day after the alleged contact may be remote, depending on the subsequent use or handling of that clothing.

More than half of all fibers used in the production of textile materials are man-made. Some man-made fibers originate from natural materials such as cotton or wood; others originate from synthetic materials. Polyester and nylon fibers are the most commonly encountered man-made fibers, followed by acrylics, rayons, and acetates. There are also many other less common man-made fibers. The amount of production of a particular man-made fiber and its end use influence the degree of rarity of a given fiber.

The shape of a man-made fiber can determine the value placed on that fiber. The cross-section of a man-made fiber can be manufacturer-specific: some cross-sections are more common than others, and some shapes may only be produced for a short period of time. Unusual cross-sections encountered through examination can add increased significance to a fiber association.

Color influences the value given to a particular fiber identification. Often several dyes are used to give a fiber a desired color. Individual fibers can be colored prior to being spun into yarns. Yarns can be dyed, and fabrics made from them can be dyed. Color can also be applied to the surface of fabric, as found in printed fabrics. How color is applied and absorbed along the length of the fiber are important comparison characteristics. Color-fading and discoloration can also lend increased value to a fiber association.

The number of fibers on the clothing of a victim identified as matching the clothing of a suspect is important in determining actual contact. The greater the number of fibers, the more likely that contact actually occurred between these individuals.

Where fibers are found also affects the value placed on a particular fiber association. The location of fibers on different areas of the body or on specific items at the crime scene influences the significance of the fiber association.

How a fabric is constructed affects the number and types of fibers that may be transferred during contact. Tightly woven or knitted fabrics shed less often than loosely knit or woven fabrics; fabrics composed of filament yarns shed less than fabrics composed of spun yarns. Certain types of fibers also tend to transfer more readily.

The age of a fabric also affects the degree of fiber transfers. Some newer fabrics may shed more readily because of an abundance of loosely adhering fibers on the surface of the fabric. Some worn fabrics may have damaged areas that easily shed fibers. Damage to a fabric caused during physical contact greatly increases the likelihood of fiber transfer.

When a questioned fiber is compared to fibers from a known fabric source, a determination is made as to whether this fiber could have originated from the known fabric. It is not possible to say positively that a fiber originated from a particular fabric, although the inability to positively associate a fiber with a source in no way diminishes the significance of a fiber association. The wide variety of fiber types, fiber colors, and fabric types can make fiber associations very significant because the value of a fiber association depends on the type of fiber, the color of the fiber, the number of fibers transferred, the location of the recovered fibers, and other factors.

It could be very helpful to know the frequency of occurrence of a particular fabric and fiber, or how many fabrics with a particular fiber type and color exist, as well as who owns them. Such information, however, is extremely difficult to obtain. If the manufacturer of a fabric is known, the possibility exists that the number of fabric units produced could also be obtained, but this information is not always available. How many garments like this still exist, and where they are located, are still in question.

Once a particular fiber of a certain type, shape, and color is produced and becomes part of a fabric, it occupies an extremely small portion of the fiber/fabric population. Exceptions to this would be white cotton fibers and blue cotton fibers like those comprising blue jeans. There are other fibers that are common, but the majority of fibers of a particular type and color constitute a very small percentage of the total number of fibers that exist in the world.

The value of the fiber associations to the Hardees shirt can be assessed by determining manufacturing information and distribution of similar shirts. It was determined that the shirts were manufactured by Westpoint Stevens, Alamac Knits in Lumberton, North Carolina specifically for the Angelica

Corporation Uniform Group and purchased by Hardees for their employees. The specific design of the shirts and limited production greatly increased the significance and relevance of the fiber associations in the case.

The shirts provided by Bell to the police were short-sleeve turquoise polo shirts. This particular shirt had been recently replaced with a multiple-color striped knit shirt and very few of the previous shirts were in circulation among Hardees employees. Angelica Corporation provided data sheets concerning specifications and standards for the shirts, and dye/production data were also provided. Samples of the Angelica fabric were provided for comparison.

An interesting aspect of the fiber comparisons in this case concerned the side-by-side comparison of a known fabric cutting of the suspect's shirt with questioned nubs recovered from the victim's items. The known cuttings failed to reveal a significant number of the nubs. Sample tapings from the surface of the suspect's shirt, however, revealed a very high population of nubs, demonstrating the importance of proper and appropriate sampling methods. It is suspected that these nubs were the result of calendaring or singeing during production.

A fabric that has just come off the loom or knitting machine is referred to as greige (pronounced "gray") goods or greige fabric; this material is not yet considered "finished." Finishing, whether chemical, mechanical, or thermal, changes a fabric's physical or chemical state. A wide variety of finishes are used to produce not only everyday consumer textiles but also for the many specialty fabrics specifically designed for health, safety, comfort, sports, and industry.

Chemical finishes may be absorbed by the fibers of a fabric (where it may or may not react with the polymer), adhere to the fiber surface, or form a coating or barrier on the fabric (Vail and Haynes 1990). Some residue from the chemical treatment may remain on the as-purchased goods. Over 3000 finishing chemicals are used on various textiles (Hochberg 1984), including resins, gums, anti-microbials, softening agents, flame retardants, and water repellents.

Mechanical finishes change the appearance or performance of a fabric through physical methods. The fabric may be flattened, crimped, or napped to produce a specific effect or look. Thermal finishes use heat to alter the fabric or fibers, either to smooth or bulk the textile. Chemical finishes, such as resins, may be set by thermal finishes as well. Table 1.1 lists the more common types of finishes (Hatch 1993: 386); of particular interest in this case are singeing and calendaring.

Singeing removes fiber ends or fibrils from a textile's surface by burning. Typically, fabrics made of cellulosic staple fibers (cotton, rayon, lyocell) will be singed in preparation for final dyeing or construction. Heated rollers or heating elements are used to burn off the fibrils as the fabric passes between or over them. Enzymes that digest cellulose are now being used to remove fibrils from cellulosic fabrics in place of singeing.

Process name	Purpose and method
Singeing or shearing	To remove protruding fibers from yarns or fabrics by passing them over a flame or heated copper plates (singeing) or by clipping (shearing), achieving a smooth fabric surface and reducing pilling propensity.
Desizing	To remove sizing (starches, gelatins, oils, waxes, and manufactured polymers such as polyvinyl alcohol, polystyrene, polyacrylic acid, and polyacetates) that was added to yarns to aid in fabric formulation by treating them in enzyme or mild alkaline solutions.
Scouring	To clean impurities and machine oils from fabrics containing cellulosic fibers by exposing them to a solution of sodium hydroxide and detergent.
Carbonizing	To eliminate plant debris from wool and specialty wool fabrics by subjecting them to sulfuric acid solutions or hydrogen chloride gas followed by heating. When the fabrics dry, the carbonized debris, which is dust-like, is removed.
Degumming	To remove the natural gum from silk fibers by boiling silk fabric in a mild alkaline solution.
Bleaching	To decolorize and remove colored matter from fabrics by exposing them to oxidizing and reducing chemicals.
Tentering	To realign yarns and extend fabrics to uniform width by using a tenter frame, a device that consists of a pair of endless chains on horizontal tracks. The fabric is held firmly at the edges by pins or clips on the chains that diverge as they advance through a heated chamber.
Calendaring	To smooth and enhance the luster of fabric surfaces, to produce a more supple hand, or to make fabrics more compact (opaque) by subjecting them to heavy pressure while they pass between two or more heavy rollers that are sometimes heated.
Decatizing	To improve hand and remove wrinkles from fabrics by circulating hot water or blowing steam through fabrics that are wound tightly on perforated rollers.

Table 1.1
Common types of finishes.

If the fabric is composed of cellulosic and synthetic, or purely synthetic fibers, singeing comes later in the finishing process. The singeing of synthetic fibers causes small molten beads, or nubs, of melted polymer to form on the surface of the fabric. The nubs interfere with the uptake of dyes and/or chemical finishes and so singeing is delayed where synthetics are involved.

Calendaring, where fabric is run between large rollers, is similar to ironing but the pressures involved are much higher. A series of rollers, which may be stacked or placed in series, compresses the fabric at pressures as high as 1 ton/in^{-2} (Hatch 1993). One or more of the rollers may be heated to produce various effects on the fabrics, typically smoothing the fabric for a more lustrous appearance and gentle drape.

While the new Hardees shirts were different in appearance to the solid blue shirts, a similar blue color was apparent in one of the stripes. Color comparison of the different colors and similar colors using microspectrophotometry revealed distinct differences in some of the colors and some similarities in one of the colors. Dye lot variations were also evident.

This case revealed the importance of conducting an organized and thorough crime scene investigation and the value of maintaining a proper focus when analyzing physical evidence in the forensic laboratory. A logical and orderly protocol for examining evidence should cover most of the important topic areas and not interfere with or destroy other analytical methods. The careful examination of vaginal and rectal swabs and fingernail scrapings for the presence of trace materials such as textile fibers can reveal valuable physical evidence. This case also highlighted the importance of a thorough and efficient processing of clothing items for trace materials prior to other laboratory testing. It also demonstrated the importance of resolving, whenever possible, the significance of matching trace evidence.

Of particular note in this case is that Everett Bell confessed to the murder of Sandra Price and to the murders of at least nine other people. Bell also admitted to five rapes in the vicinity. Although Bell has been compared to serial killers such as Ted Bundy and John Wayne Gacy, Bell's methods are even more frightening because, unlike the others, he didn't have a specific type of victim. One detective in the case stated "It didn't matter what they looked like – black, white, young, old, big, little. Any woman was a target . . . he would only take someone if he had the advantage." With a lack of patterned behavior or a victim profile to identify Bell's crimes, the trace evidence became crucial to discovering the associations between the victims and subject. It is extraordinary that a crime of this magnitude could be resolved with one of the smallest forms of physical evidence – fibers.

REFERENCES

Fiber Organon (1999) 70 (7), 107.

Hatch, K.L. (1993) *Textile Science*, Minneapolis/St Paul, MN: West Publishing.

Hochberg, E.G. (1984) *Amer. Textile Int'l*, 13 (5), 33–34, 36–39.

Vail, S.L. and Haynes, R.J., Jr (1990) "Textile Resins" in Kroschwitz, J.I., ed., *Polymers: Fibers and Technology, A Compendium.*

CHAPTER 2

WIGS AND THE SIGNIFICANCE OF ONE FIBER

Susan Ballou

INTRODUCTION

On February 17, 1970 three murders occurred and eventually Dr Jeffrey MacDonald was convicted of murdering his wife and two daughters while they lay sleeping in their beds (Potter 1995). Through all possible venues, Dr MacDonald continues to profess his innocence to these murders. He insists the murders were actually committed by a group of intruders, one of whom wore a big floppy hat, and possibly a blonde wig. In the kitchen area of the MacDonald home, evidence in the form of two long wig fibers was found entwined in the bristles of a hairbrush. Helena Stoeckley, a colonel's daughter, fit Dr MacDonald's description of one of the intruders and admitted to owning a floppy hat and blonde wig. Helena destroyed the hat and wig prior to Dr Jeffrey MacDonald's trial.

The defense contended Dr Jeffrey MacDonald's story could be corroborated with a known fiber sample from the blonde wig. This known sample would have been used as a means to evaluate the origin of the wig fibers recovered from the hairbrush, a process they were denied due to human intervention.

Wig fibers are not a common form of forensic evidence. However, when wig fibers are encountered, the composition of the recovered fibers may display characteristics that could generate valuable associative results. The quality of the wig varies considerably depending upon several factors, such as the price, end-use of the wig and the specific manufacturer. Costume wigs, for instance, display a rainbow of colors and the strands can be stiff or waxy in texture. Costume wigs are easily identified as such by visual inspection, differing significantly from wigs made for cosmetic purposes. For cosmetics, the manufacturer's goal is to produce a product that completely mimics the appearance of natural hair (Kaswell, 1995). To attain this goal, the intricacies of human hair have been studied and crafted into synthetic structures. These crafted characteristics allow a cosmetic wig strand to be easily overlooked when intermingled with human hair. In cases involving possible wig fibers, it is imperative that the examiner be diligent and methodical in the microscopic review of all submitted trace material. Omission of such scrutiny could result in failure to discover a key piece of evidence.

THE CRIME SCENE

On October 19, 1992, the police received a report of a missing woman. The woman, a recent college graduate, lived at home with her mother and had obtained employment with a business establishment in a neighboring jurisdiction. Neighbors reported they had seen her leaving for work wearing pants, trench coat and hat, the morning of October 19. The woman's failure to arrive at work instigated phone calls from her office to home, and finally to her older brother. Initial investigation of the house by the brother and responding police revealed no signs of disturbance. A flurry of speculation on her whereabouts developed during the next five days. On the fifth day, a search of a wooded area not far from the woman's home resulted in the recovery of a bloody pillow and pillowcase. This discovery changed the direction and focus of the investigation.

The fabric and design of the pillowcase matched remaining linens located in the woman's bedroom. According to the mother, the condition of the bedroom was typical (Figure 2.1). The bed covers were disheveled and the room was

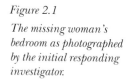

Figure 2.1

The missing woman's bedroom as photographed by the initial responding investigator.

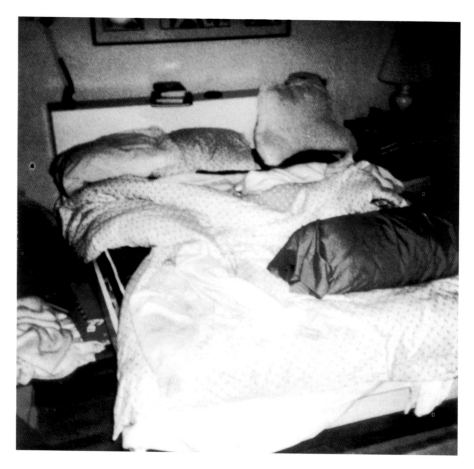

relatively cluttered with clothing, pillows and dust present on the floor. However, an examination of the bed revealed that both mattress pad and fitted sheet were missing. The remaining bed linens along with other potential evidentiary items were removed from the room for laboratory submission. Forensic examination of the mattress revealed three small circular bloodstains at the head of the mattress and a long narrow bloodstain on the right seam edge. To obtain more information about the amount of blood present the chemical test, luminol, was used. Luminol is a chemical mixture that produces a luminescence when in contact with blood or with other products, such as metals or cleaning agents (Grispino 1990). Although Luminol may react with other compounds, due to its sensitivity it is a valuable searching tool for minute traces of blood. When this test was conducted on the mattress, luminescence was present across the top and along the right side of the bed, a pattern consistent with the normal sleeping position of the victim. Continuation of the luminol test through the house uncovered no additional bloodstains. Dogs, given the scent of the pillowcase in the wooded area, led their handlers through residential backyards and streets to the back door of the missing woman's house.

A name arose that was familiar to the assigned investigators after further discussions with the missing woman's mother. While describing a man she employed as a part-time gardener, the investigators were shocked to find this individual had been a suspect in the disappearance of a six-year-old girl years earlier. The girl had never been found, and at that time there was not enough evidence to strongly implicate him with her disappearance.

With a possible suspect, investigators obtained search warrants and discovered startling information that this man had made his move days prior to the woman's disappearance. A receipt from a local hardware store listed a purchase of three rolls of duct tape, braided rope and mason line. The materials were paid from his personal checking account with the missing woman's name written in the memo space on the check. Another receipt dated October 19, the first day of her disappearance, was from a department store, for a white queen-size fitted sheet. The size of the sheet was too large for any of his mattresses, but just right to replace the missing sheet from the victim's bed. Cancelled checks directed the investigators to rental storage lockers. Documents at this facility noted he had visited these locations during the first few days after the woman's disappearance. One of the lockers was located in a state approximately 450 miles away, near where his grandparents' graves were located. The cemetery caretaker had seen an individual that matched the suspect's description after the woman's disappearance. Oddly enough, the ground near the grandparents' grave had recently been disturbed. Careful filtering and examination of the disturbed ground by the investigators revealed no indication of body fluid seepage into the surrounding area and no fragments of clothing, tissue, or hair.

In the laboratory, analysis began on the submitted evidence. The pillowcase and pillow were examined for trace evidence yielding a few head hairs. The items were examined for the identification of the apparent bloodstains. Through documentation on the missing woman and known blood samples from the immediate family members, the pillowcase stains were shown to have genetic conformity with the missing woman's mother and brother.

Once the stains on an item or garment are noted, recorded and removed for testing, the item is usually packaged, sealed, and released for storage. However, the location of the pillow and pillowcase, and the number of varied bloodstains on these items were intriguing. The next few days were spent subjecting the pillowcase to various light sources, re-marking folds and scrutinizing each obscure detail. Hidden in a corner of the pillowcase were faint patterns in blood, part of a patent print (Figure 2.2). The print was barely visible. A protein stain, Amido Black, was used to enhance the print making the print suitable for fingerprint examination (Police Scientific Development Branch 1986). Evidence originating from the missing person would be expected on the pillowcase if the pillowcase were in fact part of the missing woman's bed linens. The odds that this print would match up with the missing woman's were favorable. However, this was not the case. The suspect's fingerprints were already on file in the automated fingerprint identification system from a prior arrest. The enhanced print from the pillowcase resulted in a "hit". Visual verification by two independent fingerprint examiners confirmed the print as originating from the part-time gardener.

This was thought to be the needed link in the investigation. However, the suspect's attorneys explained to the media that their client lived out of his truck and would regularly park in the nearby parking lot, where the pillowcase and pillow were found. He would routinely walk through the woods and occasionally pick up abandoned goods to see if they were usable, discarding them if they were not. The defense contended this must have occurred with the pillow and pillowcase, resulting with the suspect unknowingly leaving his print in the damp liquid on the fabric. Understanding the plausible nature of this explanation and the requirement for the prosecution to prove beyond a reasonable doubt, laboratory examination continued.

Of the remaining physical evidence submitted to the crime laboratory, the majority proved of little value in discovering a link between the gardener and the disappearance of the woman. Bloodstains found on items taken from his campsite were unsuitable for examination. Other bloodstains found on his bed linens were identified through DNA analysis as being his blood. These types of results continued for the next several months; the woman still had not been located.

It was expected that trial would commence, even with the limited physical

(a)

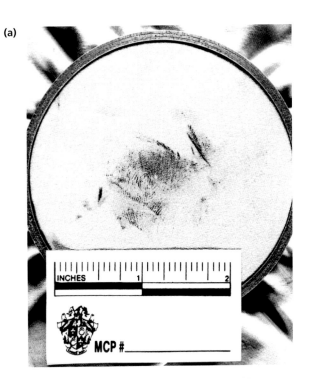

Figure 2.2
Enhanced fingerprint (a)
found on the pillowcase
(b).

(b)

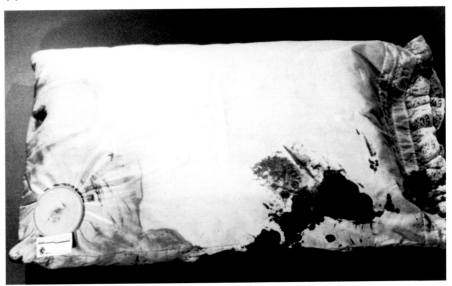

evidence. The majority of the case would be testimony from various individuals armed with suggestive statements made by the suspect. In the remaining time prior to the trial, portions of evidence had yet to be examined, specifically the collected hair samples. Known samples of the woman's head hair were recovered from the two hairbrushes she had on her dresser, and from a brush removed from the glove compartment of her car. Gross examination showed the hairs from each brush to be consistent with one another. Out of 90 hairs removed from the brushes, a representative sample of 30 hairs were measured and mounted for examination. Cursory microscopic review of the selected known hairs revealed an unexpected observation. One of the selected head hairs was in fact a synthetic wig fiber (Figure 2.3). Through additional testing the fiber was identified as modified acrylonitrile, more commonly termed, modacrylic (Grieve and Cabiness 1985). This wig fiber had been recovered from one of the two hairbrushes found on top of her dresser. Microscopic examination of the remaining mounted hairs, the additional known hairs and the large number of questioned hairs recovered from the house interior revealed no additional synthetic wig fibers.

The investigators were supplied with this new information and subsequent inquiries provided several facts. No one in the missing woman's family or her close friends owned or wore wigs. Due to the woman's height, finding dress pants of suitable length was difficult; therefore, she never wore pants to work, a detail in conflict with the description of interviewed neighbor during the first day of her disappearance. These details now cast doubt as to the identity of the individual leaving the house the morning of October 19. Additional searches of the suspect's local storage facility produced a hat, trench coat, pants, and 24 wigs and wiglets. All of the wigs and wiglets were submitted to the crime laboratory for comparison with the one modacrylic fiber from the crime scene. Through visual and microscopic comparisons the majority of the wigs and wiglets were eliminated as the source of the modacrylic fiber (SWGMAT 1998:

Figure 2.3

Recovered wig fiber from the missing woman's hairbrush.

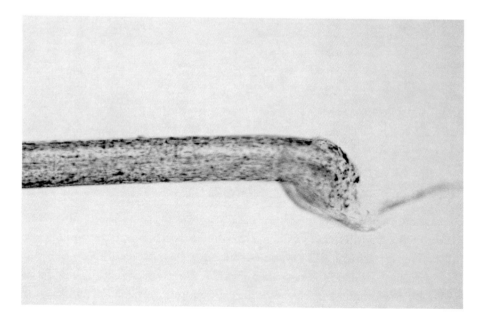

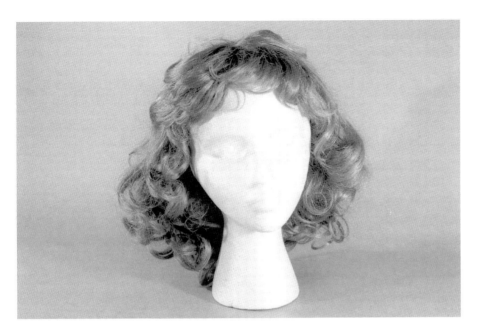

Figure 2.4

*Of the 24 wigs and wiglets
recovered from the
suspect's storage facility,
this wig matched the
single wig fiber.*

11–23). One wig, by a major manufacturer, exhibited all of the same optical characteristics as the questioned wig fiber (Figure 2.4). The modacrylic fiber and the selected wig were submitted to the Hairs and Fibers Unit[1] of the FBI laboratory in Washington, DC for additional classification. The dye composition was classified using a Zeiss MPM-400 microspectrophotometer. This instrument has the capability to discern between the numerous commercial dyes that were used in the United States at the time of this event. Through patents, each company documents dye formulations of slightly different characteristics providing a vast array of colors advantageous to forensic analysis. Subjecting the crime scene fiber to this examination, a spectrum of its color was produced, matching it specifically to the selected wig (Figure 2.5).

At the crime laboratory, the tedious task of comparing the vast number of questioned hairs to the known samples from the suspect and from the hairbrushes was conducted. After days of microscopic examination, one head hair fragment consistent with the known hairbrush samples was found on a sheet recovered from the back of the suspect's truck. From the more than 150 hairs recovered from her bedroom, one head hair was found to be consistent with the suspect's.

On June 14, 1993, the part-time gardener plea-bargained to a reduced charge of murder in the second degree with the stipulation he must reveal the location of the body. He directed the investigators to a shallow grave not far from where he had staked an elaborate campsite. When the body was uncovered, bits of duct tape were found stuck in the remaining strands of hair. The condition of the body was prohibitive for determination of the exact cause

[1] Now the Trace Evidence Unit.

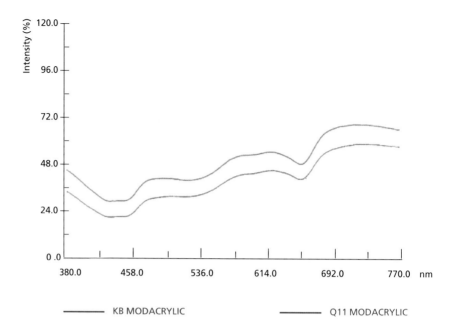

Figure 2.5

Visible spectra from the wig fiber (Q11) and the recovered wig (K8).

of death as reflected in the medical examiner's certificate of death "cutting wound of neck and possibly suffocation" as the mode of death. The part-time gardener was sentenced to 30 years in the State Penitentiary.

ANALYSIS

Thorough documentation is critical for the analysis and interpretation of physical evidence. Details that seem evident may mentally disappear from the examiner's mind if not promptly and thoroughly recorded. An examiner understands the imperative nature of this task when dealing with transient evidence such as fibers and hairs.

Recently deposited hairs or fibers may remain on the top of the surface they land on. Depending upon the circumstances of the case, how the hair or fiber was found may allow an examiner to provide an estimated time frame for the occurrence of events (Robertson 1992). The examiner must take into consideration that hairs or fibers can become embedded or moved with the surrounding environment over time. Fibers or hairs on a carpeted surface are a perfect example of how deposited evidence will lay on the surface of the carpet initially and then become embedded into the carpet after withstanding the force of repeated walking or movement. On tiled or wood floors dust may accumulate around deposited hairs or fibers creating a mass of trace evidence continually growing in size.

One of the most important aspects of initial control over the crime scene is to preserve the scene with minimal contamination and disturbance of physical evidence (FBI 1992). This was not a viable option in the above-described homicide scenario, due to the fact that the direction of the investigation had not been determined until almost five days after the murder took place. Several investigators, the missing woman's family members, and friends had intruded upon the bedroom. Still, upon entrance into the bedroom, initial assessment included oblique lighting to locate any fibers or hairs for manual recovery. Located hairs or fibers were recovered using tweezers and deposited into sterile metal tins. The tins were labeled according to time, date, collector's initials and area of recovery. Once manual recovery was complete, removable items in the bedroom that warranted further examination such as the throw pillows, comforter, bed sheets, and clothing were labeled, packaged and sealed for transport to the crime laboratory.

In the laboratory, analysis of the submitted evidence is an extension of the crime scene search, progressing from the basic search techniques to scientific elaboration. At all times thorough documentation must accompany each action. The pillows, bed linens, comforter and clothing were individually examined over clean exam tables covered with clean white paper. Trace evidence, visually located, was recovered with forceps and placed into labeled sterile tins. Each item, the pillows, bed linens, etc., were then taped or scraped to recover additional evidence. Once recovery was complete, each taping or collected tin was subjected to macroscopic examination (Robertson 1992).

The process applied to the hairbrush for the recovery of the synthetic wig fiber occurred in relatively the same fashion. Statements from the woman's mother and girlfriends established that the hairbrushes were in fact the missing woman's, thereby supporting the basis for using the brushes as a known source of hair. The style, brand, size and color of each hairbrush were documented. Then using forceps, the hairs were removed from the bristles over a clean sheet of white paper (SWGMAT 1998: 1–8). Measurements were conducted using a metric ruler and then independently holding each hair taught over the cali-brated surface. Using forceps, the same hair was then viewed under the stereo-microscope for estimation of gross characteristics, subsequent examination was prepared by placing the hairs on a microscope slide with mounting medium and cover slip. Each slide was labeled and numbered according to the selected identifiers for that particular hair as documented in the case notes. When more than one hair was mounted per slide, an established system was used to allow individual identification, and to allow for corresponding reference for each hair to case notes (Gaudette 1985). The mounted hairs were then examined in detail on a single stage of the comparison microscope using 200×–400× magni-fication. The information obtained was recorded in case notes on a prepared form listing characteristic categories.

The microscopic revelation of the synthetic wig fiber changed the direction of the examination from hairs to fibers. Using a stage micrometer, the diameter of the fiber was calculated along with documentation of color, striation, delusterants and imperfections (Grieve and Griffin 1999). These characteristics were used to evaluate a possible match with the submitted 24 wigs and wiglets that had been recovered from the storage facility. Although many agencies have spectral instrumentation available for fiber analysis, the microscope should always be the first step. At this point, microscopic evaluation may provide sufficient information to eliminate the fiber as having originated from the suspected source. Color hue is a subjective feature; however, common sense will permit the elimination of a reddish brown wig fiber from originating from an ash blonde wig (SWGMAT 1998: 11–25). The open stage of the stereomicroscope provided a means to view large portions of each wig, allowing quick characterization and verification of color consistency within the wig or wiglet. This process eliminated all but three wigs that were subsequently subjected to analysis using comparison microscopy. Numerous fibers were removed from each of the suspected wigs in order to determine characteristic consistency between the fibers of each wig. No gross variations were noted with only one wig exhibiting the same internal characteristics as the crime scene wig fiber.

Chemical composition was determined using the Nicolet Fourier Transform Infrared spectrometer (FTIR) with microscope attachment (Nic-Plan). A fiber, consistent in internal microscopic characteristics as the crime scene fiber, was selected from the associative wig. Manipulating a small cutting of this fiber through stereoscopic methods, the cutting was flattened on a microscopic slide surface with a roller knife. Still working under the stereoscope, the razor knife tip of the roller knife was then used to lift the minute section onto a diamond window already in place inside a compression cell metal holder (Gal *et al.* 1991). The other diamond window was placed on top of the prepared sample and the circular metal top was manually screwed in place. Although the use of the micro-compression diamond cell unit provides crushing and flattening of hard materials without the prior preparation by a roller wheel, additional flattening techniques have demonstrated improved spectra results. The diamond cell windows also provide a large working area, suitable for accommodating multiple samples. Placing the compression cell on the stage of the Nic-Plan, the apertures were positioned to ensure capture of an area of the fiber that demonstrated compositional uniformity. The remaining analysis steps were controlled through computer software programs. After subtracting out background interference, the resulting spectra were searched against several installed libraries, which identified the fiber as modacrylic (Tungol *et al.* 1991). After tool and instrument surfaces were cleaned that had come into direct contact to the selected wig fiber, the crime scene fiber was subjected to the same protocol (SWGMAT 1998: 11–23).

To relate specifically the crime scene fiber to the selected wig, further characterization was conducted and one obvious area was color. Colors can vary in such subtle hues and the vast array of dye possibilities is enormous. Visible spectroscopy of fibers is an objective method for the determination of dye composition (Eyring 1994). The crime scene fiber and the selected wig expressed suitable dye levels and conformity for this procedure. The fibers were examined with a Zeiss MPM-400 microspectrophotometer at the FBI Laboratory in the visible range (380–770 nm) at 12V with a tungsten source.

INTERPRETATION

Each step in the tier of analysis provides compounding information on the characteristics of a fiber. When the totality of the garnered information is compared to the information obtained from a known source, the similarity between a questioned and a known sample can provide scientific basis for "possible same source origin". In contrast to the strength of a similarity, the moment a difference is found between the known fiber and the unknown fiber which cannot be scientifically supported, a non-match is declared eliminating the need for further examinations (SWGMAT 1998: 1–8).

In this homicide case, the synthetic qualities of the crime scene wig fiber were determined when the comparison microscope was utilized. There may have been some speculation that this particular strand produced a higher sheen than the other hairs during the gross examination with the stereomicroscope. However, the possibility of a synthetic fiber being present among head hairs was not anticipated. The main objective was to initiate a known profile of the missing woman's hair characteristics. Therefore, the basic characteristics were documented and the next tier was tackled, comparison microscopy. The increased magnification of the comparison microscope and a suitable mountant allowed easy identification of the synthetic fiber (Smith 1990). The microscopic examination included the physical characteristics of the fiber such as denier, color, and delusterants: their size, shape and distribution (Saferstein 1981). Notation was made of any external layer imperfections such as micropores and "fish-eye" markings (Grieve and Griffin 1999). The total sum of these microscopic characteristics was shown to be the same between the one crime scene fiber and to the one wig. These similar factors were not yet strong enough to support the weight of "same source origin".

FTIR provides an easy method to identify the organic components of a substance. The collection of absorption bands are interpreted to determine the composition of the sample and then used to find a comparable match with reference samples (Tungol *et al.* 1991). In forensic drug chemistry, these features comprise the "fingerprint" identification of a suspected drug. Each type of drug will produce its own unique set of spectral fingerprints. This is also true for the identification of the polymer or copolymer in fiber analysis; a specific polymer will provide its own unique spectral fingerprint and in this case generic class (Kirkbride 1992). However, polymer composition is just the start for fiber manufactures. Once the fiber polymer is selected the solid proceeds through numerous steps in the manufacturing process, each step adding additional characteristics. This infers that the identification of the polymer composition is not unique for "same source origin", but has provided a class characterization of the fiber.

The color determination of the crime scene fiber and the selected wig fibers added another comparative aspect in the tier of analysis. The microspectrophotometer measures the amount of colored light an object reflects or transmits (Eyring 1994). The visible range scanned was 380 nm to 770 nm producing an absorbance spectra. A comparison between the two resulting spectra was presented by sequentially plotting them on the same chart followed by evaluation of peak intensity, width and position. A visual evaluation was conducted on all absorbance values. These values must be identical before a positive association can be attributed to the samples. The spectra must also produce a range in values, not a flat line, so that the resulting peaks provide enough variation to show the fiber actually reflected color.

At the completion of the visible spectroscopy analysis the crime scene wig fiber and the selected wig fiber exhibited the color in the visible range. To interpret the strength of this result, an examiner must have knowledge of other factors. First, the examiner should be aware of manufacturer procedures. Trade secrets are a high security issue and patent applications are not always submitted since they require detailed research information to be divulged. The extensive information submitted with the patent application will eventually become public knowledge providing guidance for another firm to make their own product version for profit. However, if a manufacturer has a patent on a particular formula, product blueprint or protocol, then an item characterized as exhibiting the patented information can be directly associated to the company holding the patent license. In this homicide scenario, because the microspectrophotometer results confirmed that the wavelength characteristics of the crime scene wig fiber could be superimposed on the known wig fiber spectra, then the crime scene modacrylic fiber could be associated to the particular manufacturer. Although these results produced a strong associative value, this value remains a class characteristic.

The combination of all comparable physical attributes for both fibers generated a strong associative probability (SWGMAT 1998: 1–8). Added emphasis should be made that no discrepancies were found between the fiber recovered from the hairbrush and the fibers composing the known wig. In the course of this comparison, the product label of the known wig, 100 per cent modacrylic, had been verified. The examination process eliminated all of the other submitted wigs as possible contributors to the crime-scene wig fiber. Therefore, other manufactures can be eliminated as possible sources, which in effect reduces the volume of potential wigs. To continually narrow the possibilities from class to individualizing, additional questions should be investigated such as: the number of wigs manufactured by the identified company, the number of modacrylic wigs produced, of this number how many wigs had the identified dye and the measured fiber length, and finally, the number of wigs sold in the United States (particularly in the general geographical area). Without this information, the tone of the interpretation statement should embrace the following; the crime scene wig fiber (item *x*) originated from a particular manufacturer and is consistent in all respects with the fiber composition of the submitted wig (item *y*) bearing the same manufacturer's label.

The physical information does not support a statement that the fiber did in fact originate from the known wig. Adding production statistics can provide a clearer view of the random possible occurrence for this particular wig and a means to reach beyond class characteristics.

WIGS AND THEIR MANUFACTURE

Wig fashion, the vain attempt to restore past grandeur, started in the early 17th century (Maginnis 2000). It appears that even at this time premature baldness was a malady borne by men. In 1624, while still fairly young, King Louis XIII became bald. To hide this unfortunate occurrence he wore wigs and started a fashion craze that would sweep the European nobility. These wigs were constructed of horsehair, yak hair and human hair and were heavily powdered with starch to maintain the desirable lighter look. Wig fashion extended over to the New World and prominent men such as John Adams and Patrick Henry were depicted in history books wearing the "bob" or "short tie" wig. The wig fetish was brought to a halt during the 1790s through government intervention on two fronts. The British, eager to tax anything and everything, placed a tax on the needed hair powder thereby squashing demand. The association made by the French people was slightly more life-threatening. The wig was seen as a symbol of the reigning aristocrats and at that time in history any association with them could bring death.

The advent of synthetic hair fibers dramatically changed the wig market. Wigs were now affordable and could be manufactured in a vast array of colors (Kaswell 1995). Wig manufacturers used a single component or a blend of synthetic fibers such as nylon, polyester, polypropylene, modacrylic and vinyon. However, the features of some fibers did little to emulate the desirable qualities of human hair. The brassy colors and stiff texture were attributable to nylon and polyester fibers. Fiber manufacturers had yet to figure out how to reproduce the delustering effect that human hair scales exhibit naturally (Kaswell 1995). Improvements in the manufacturing of synthetic fibers have gained respect for the synthetic hair wig.

Polyester, introduced in the United States in 1953 by DuPont, was very strong, resistant to stretching and resistant to chemicals (American Fiber Manufacturers Association 2000c). This would not do for a product that would have to succumb to curling and chemical processing such as permanents. To make the fiber more pliable the manufacturing procedure included subjecting the fiber to sodium hydroxide. Through this chemical process pitting was created in the fiber surface allowing flexibility (Kaswell 1995). By chance, this action creating the pliable nature also created a delustering effect to the polyester fiber surface.

Due to its very shiny appearance, nylon did not enter into the arena for wig production until late in the 20th century (Kaswell 1995). Research with the fiber at that time proposed methods for producing indentations or etching into the nylon fiber surface after the melt spinning step (American Fiber Manufacturers Association 2000d). Spinning is a term referring to the technique where the polymer is forced through tiny holes in an object called the spinneret and the newly formed strands are allowed to solidify. There are four methods for spinning, wet, dry, melt and get; the differences between them depend upon the state of the polymer prior to entering the spinneret and the method of solidification after. Melt spinning refers to the method where melting of the polymer occurs prior to forcing through the spinneret followed by direct cooling after extrusion. To obtain the desired surface features on nylon fibers the melt spin method was modified to require the extruded filaments to enter into a higher than 30°C water bath, remaining immersed for the length of time determined by process parameters (Kaswell 1995).

The most common wig fiber, modacrylic, is a copolymer of acrylonitrile mixed with other constituents (Grieve and Griffin 1999). The Federal Trade Commission (FTC) defines a modacrylic fiber as having a composition of acrylonitrile units greater or equal to 35 per cent or less than 85 per cent by mass (American Fiber Manufacturers Association 2000a). This wide range of acrylonitrile units allows incredible latitude for manufactures to vary the production of modacrylic fibers into a variety of products. However, for wig production, the manufacturers tend not to vary the acrylonitrile content since the greater the number of acrylonitrile units, the greater the fiber strength and thermal stability (Grieve and Griffin 1999). Even taking this into consideration, modacrylic fibers still fall behind polyester and nylon for softening and melting temperatures (Kaswell 1995). Modacrylic fibers soften at 160°C and melt at 190°C, compared to polyester fibers which soften at 235°C and melt at 250°C.

The FTIR spectra reflects the mass to unit ratio of the acrylonitrile present in the modacrylic fiber, providing possible variance between different manufacturers' fibers (Grieve and Griffin 1999) – see Figures 2.6 to 2.16.[2]

In a pure liquid state, acrylonitrile is a flammable and explosive compound. With a boiling point of 77°C, acrylonitrile can produce toxic effects similar to cyanide poisoning (NIOSH 1997). Depending upon the purpose of the fiber, the acrylonitrile is copolymerized with a varying range of other compounds, such as vinyl bromide, vinyl chloride, vinylidene chloride and terpolymers (Grieve and Griffin 1999). The addition of aromatic or aliphatic compounds assist in the acceptance of dyes and the incorporation of esters also affect fiber shrinkage.

Modacrylic fibers are either wet spun or dry spun (American Fiber Manufacturers Association 2000a). Wet spun refers to resins dissolved in solvent and extruded directly into a chemical bath. Dry spun also requires the resin to be dissolved in a solvent but the extruded fibers are subjected to a flow of air instead of a bath (American Fiber Manufacturers Association 2000d). The air contact evaporates off the solvent thereby solidifying the fiber. If the resin is not completely dissolved prior to extrusion, the process itself produces characteristic wig markings. Incomplete or undissolved resin polymer produces markings or imperfections, called "fish-eye" or micropores that are readily recognizable with the aid of a microscope (Grieve and Griffin 1999). Since these markings exist due to the general manufacturing process, they are not limited to a single manufacturer. Most other inclusions such as pigment or inorganic compounds (e.g. antimony trioxide) are used to meet a specified requirement, either to increase the flame resistance or increase delustering effects in the final product.

Each fiber type portrays its own desirable property for consideration in the production of wigs. Nylon and polyester have high melting temperatures compared to modacrylic and therefore can withstand the heat intensity of curling irons (Kaswell 1995). Polypropylene is very resistant to moisture and chemicals, qualities that can be desirable in wig maintenance but difficult to work with during the addition of dyes (American Fiber Manufacturers Association 2000b). To compensate for this characteristic, manufacturers must pre-select the fiber color and add it directly to the polymerization step or during melt spinning. Modacrylic and vinyon (polyvinyl chloride) both soften at low temperatures; this feature allows the molding and embossing of the fibers to take on features desirable to mimic human hair. These attributes add another delustering step toward the reduction of the natural glare produced by synthetic fibers.

A few corporations were contacted regarding the current manufacturing of fibers for wig production. DuPont – "The miracles of science" – has never

[2] Various fiber samples were collected and prepared for digital photography; a few of these samples were also subjected to spectral analysis using a Perkin-Elmer FTIR with SpectroTech microscope attachment. Scans were conducted in the reflectance mode and recorded from 4000 to 500 cm^{-1}, with a resolution setting of 2. The digital imaging was conducted using an Olympus BH2 microscope with Fuji Camera attachment.

Figure 2.6
Kaneka Corporation,
modacrylic fiber
(Kanekalon) with corre-
sponding FTIR spectra.

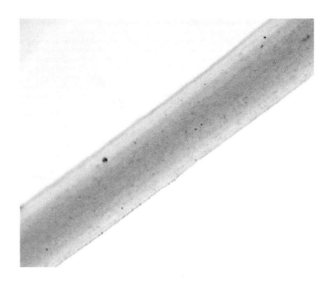

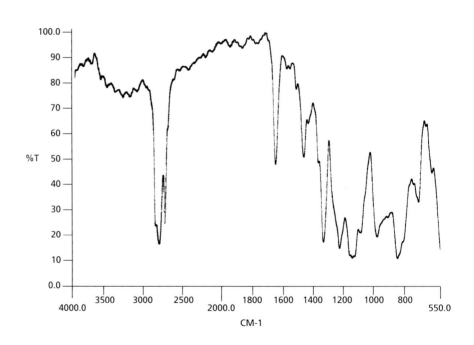

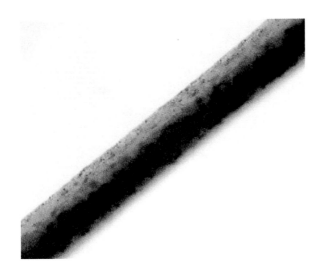

Figure 2.7
Unknown manufacturer,
modacrylic wig fiber with
corresponding FTIR
spectra.

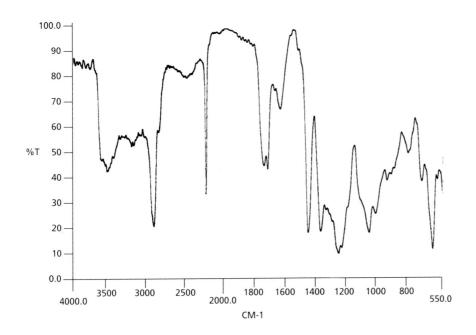

Figure 2.8

Mattel Inc. 1976 Barbie Doll hair, brown color, with corresponding FTIR spectra.

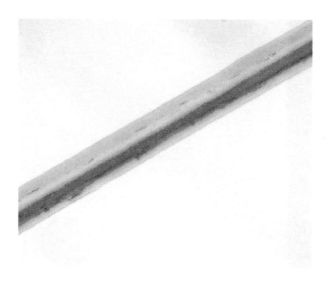

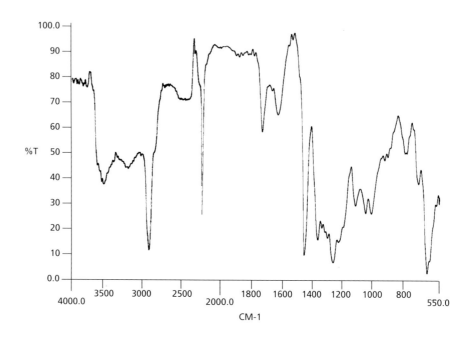

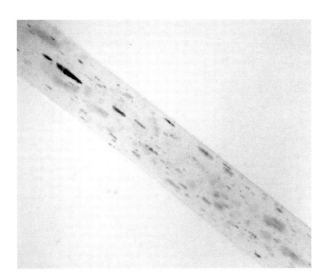

Figure 2.9
Clown costume wig,
polypropylene fiber with
corresponding FTIR
spectra.

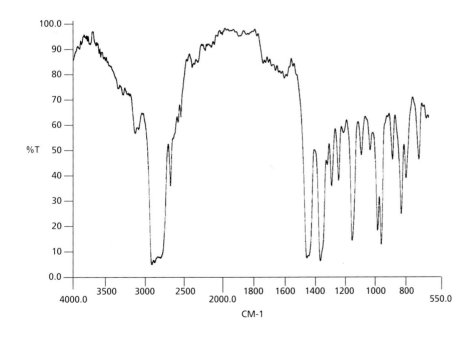

Figure 2.10
Union Carbide,
modacrylic fiber (Dynel),
from an Eva Gabor wig
with corresponding FTIR
spectra.

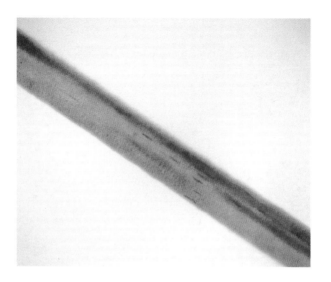

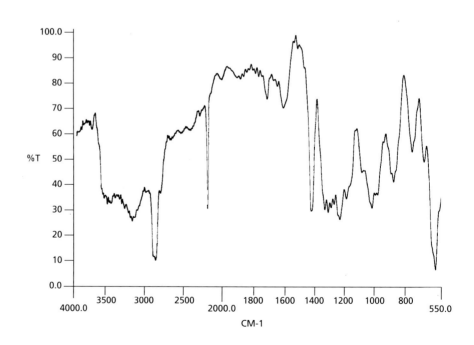

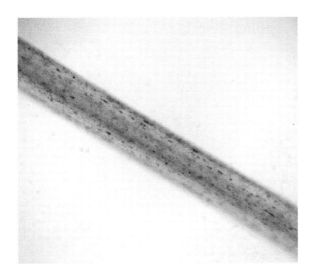

Figure 2.11
Kaneka Corporation,
modacrylic fiber
(Kanekalon Blend), from
a Paula Young wig with
corresponding FTIR
spectra.

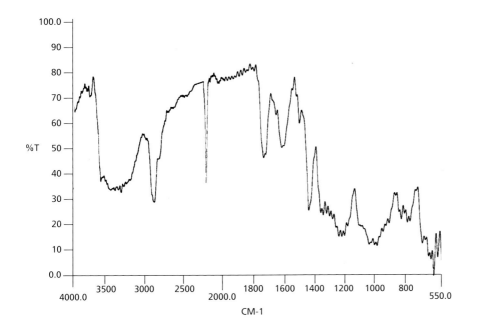

Figure 2.12
Monsanto, modacrylic
fiber (Elura blend)

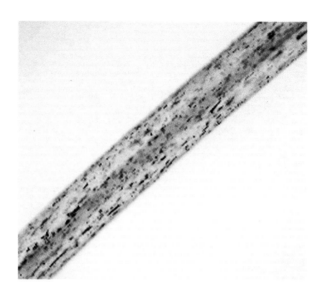

Figure 2.13
Kaneka Corporation,
modacrylic fiber
(Kanekalon + QTEK)
from a Rene of Paris wig.

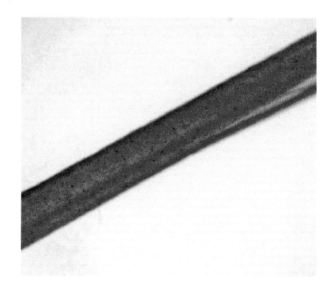

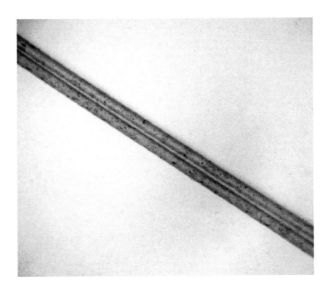

Figure 2.14
Kaneka Corporation,
modacrylic fiber
(Kanekalon SF)

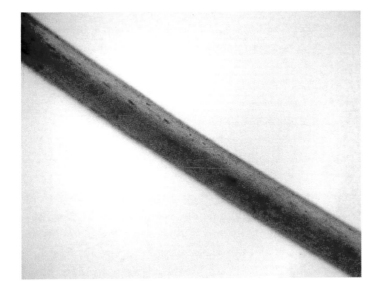

Figure 2.15
Kaneka Corporation,
modacrylic fiber
(Kanekalon 7)

Figure 2.16
Monsanto, modacrylic
fiber (Elura #27).

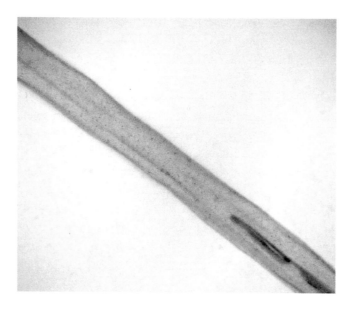

produced modacrylic fibers for wig use. Union Carbide was the first to commercialize modacrylic fiber production in 1949 and no longer offers this product. Monsanto, now called Solutia, used to produce wig fibers (Elura and SEF). In 1977 Solutia sold the wig fiber manufacturing side of the business to Alkinco of New York, NY. Elura and SEF both contain vinyl bromide and vinylidene chloride in their composition and chemically differ in dye sites. Kaneka is the largest supplier of modacrylic fibers; their manufacturing plant is in Osaka, Japan. The bulk fibers are then sent to Korea for wig production. Kaneka Corporation currently produces a number of different fibers to meet client specification:

- Kanekalon S or 7 general wigs
- Kanekalon 2, fine fiber requirement
- Kanekalon 3, for braiding or soft texture
- Kanekalon Z, for hair weaves or mixed with human hair

Kaneka Corporation briefly described their wig manufacturing process. Kanekalon polymer liquid contains acrylonitrile, vinyl chloride, and vinyl acetate with other components and is dyed after the filaments are formed through wet spinning. When the filaments are dyed in this fashion it is called "tow" dyed. The dyed filaments are measured and cut; these varying length filament bundles are referred to as "length of the tow". Different colors of "length of tow" are collected for formation of a single wig and hackling blends the fibers. Hackling is the procedure of repeatedly drawing the bundle of fibers over a large metal toothcomb. This action produces subtle color hues by intermingling the complementarily-colored fibers. Besides blending colors, hackling is also used to blend different fiber types. A wig with a label marked as 80 per cent modacrylic and 20 per cent vinyon is referring to the percentage composition of modacrylic fibers mixed with vinyon fibers, not a fiber polymer bicomponent. Once the tow and fiber composition has been selected, the blended fibers are sewn together into a long strip called a weft. The weft is conditioned then placed on paper sheets and rolled onto aluminum pipes. The pipes vary in diameter, and the diameter selection depends on the desired tightness of the curl. Once rolled, the pipes are placed into large ovens to set the curl. The curled strips are removed from the pipes ready for machine stitching onto a wig cap structure. Hand-tied wig construction follows the described protocol except that it eliminates the machine-stitching steps.

SUMMARY

It is very important that the examiner understands the boundaries of analysis and how to present the full extent of these results during testimony. Many expert witnesses rely too heavily on the prosecution to ask or phrase the appropriate questions, when it is the expert who has the freedom to expound on the facts. Unfortunately, jurors may give too much weight to the only interpretation offered because the expert neglected to expound beyond the limited scope of the question proffered by the prosecution. The assurance of an unbiased testimony results when the expert takes it upon himself or herself to supply other perfectly viable scenarios regarding the questioned evidence. In this regard the inclusion of production statistics would provide added information the jury could use to weigh up the strength of the one wig fiber. Although all of the physical properties revealed class characteristics, the expert should emphasize the number of attributes identified were also present in the known sample.

In homicides or missing persons cases, where a body is not available for recovery of known samples, investigators, crime scene personnel, and forensic examiners must be keenly aware of all avenues for obtaining references. The presented case demonstrated the importance of the collection of the hairbrushes from the victim's dresser and vehicle glove compartment. If the brushes had been overlooked, and not recovered and examined, the vital key to solving this case would have been lost. The wig fiber, the one piece of evidence providing the missing clue for unraveling how events took place, would never have been found. Armed with this additional information, the Assistant State's Attorney prepared the following time line to the occurrence of events surrounding the homicide case.

In early October, the suspect purchased his listed items from the local hardware store in anticipation of the mother departing on a scheduled trip thereby leaving the woman home alone. One Sunday evening, knowing the location of the hidden spare key, he entered the house through the back door. Death was initiated through suffocation shown by the lack of spurious blood in the bedroom. Duct tape was wrapped around the woman's head and scissors were used on the neck and ears perhaps to remove jewelry. This resulted in a flow of blood. The woman was then "mummified" in the mattress pad and fitted sheet along with other bloodstained items, including the pillow with pillowcase. This limited any further bloodstaining inside the house. She was apparently carried out the back door and through the darkened neighborhood, then the suspect stopped for a rest. While waiting to see or hear if anyone was following he failed to notice the dropped pillow and pillowcase. He then moved toward his truck in the nearby parking lot to leave.

Early the next morning he returned to the house to eliminate any speculation on her disappearance. Using the woman's bedroom, the suspect dressed to mimic the activities expected during her normal workday. Not realizing the woman normally wore skirts, he had brought pants and a trench coat in an effort to provide the most coverage, his first uncalculated mistake. Checking his appearance in her bedroom mirror he made final adjustments to the wig he had selected. Using one of the hairbrushes on the dresser top, he brushed the wig strands in place, his second mistake. Carrying her briefcase, he then walked out into the crisp fall morning air to establish the pretense of her heading off to work. Returning to his campsite to change he then drove to a department store and purchased a bed sheet. He had intended to replace the fitted sheet and properly make up the bed so no one would know exactly when, where and how her disappearance occurred. This was never accomplished since the woman's brother, accompanied by a friend, had already been notified of his sister's failure to show up for work and had started to canvas the neighborhood. Recognizing the approaching vehicle as belonging to the part-time gardener the brother tried to stop him for possible information. In a panic, the suspect turned his vehicle around and sped away keeping the newly purchased white fitted sheet in the bed of his truck.

Various items belonging to the victim were recovered from hidden stashes buried on his family's property. It is speculated that the grandparents' gravesite held some of these trophies as well as tokens from other victims, prompting the suspect to move them when the investigation started to close in on him.

ACKNOWLEDGEMENTS

The author would like to thank the American Society for Testing and Materials (ASTM), 1916 Race Street, Philadelphia, PA 19103 for authorized reprint from the Journal of Forensic Sciences, July 1995; David Exline of Chemicon, Pennsylvania (previously with RJ Lee Group, Pennsylvania, during his assistance) for his time and skill with the spectral and digital representation of the selected fibers, and Glenn Schubert with the Illinois State Police for supplying a majority of the featured fibers.

REFERENCES

American Fiber Manufacturers Association (2000a) *Fibersource*. Available at http://www.fibersource.com/f-tutor/modacrylic.htm

American Fiber Manufacturers Association (2000b) *Fibersource*. Available at http://www.fibersource.com/f-tutor/olefin.htm

American Fiber Manufacturers Association (2000c) *Fibersource*. Available at http://www.fibersource.com/f-tutor/prods.htm

American Fiber Manufacturers Association (2000d) *Fibersource*. Available at http://www.fibersource.com/f-tutor/techpag.htm

Eyring, M.B. (1994) *Analytica Chimica Acta*, 288, 25–34.

FBI (1992) *Handbook of Forensic Science, Collection, Identification and Shipping Index*, Washington, DC: Federal Bureau of Investigation.

Gal, T., Ambrus, I. and Urazu, S. (1991) *Acta Chim. Hung.*, 128, 919–928.

Gaudette, B.D. (1985) *Crime Laboratory Digest*, 12, 44–59.

Grieve, M.C. and Cabiness, L.R. (1985) *Forensic Science International*, 29, 129–146.

Grieve, M.C. and Griffin. R.M.E. (1999) *Scientific & Technical*, 39, 151–162.

Grispino, R.R.J. (1990) *Crime Laboratory Digest*, 17, 13–23.

Kaswell, E.R. (1995) *Textile Chemists and Colorists*, 27, 21–24.

Kirkbride, K.P. (1992) *Forensic Examination of Fibres*, ed. J. Robertson, pp. 181–218. New York: Ellis Horwood.

Maginnis, T. (2000) *18th Century Hair and Wigs*. Available at http://www.costumes.org/pages/18thhair.htm

National Institute for Occupational Safety and Health (NIOSH) (1997) *Current 18 Acrylonitrile*. Available at http://www.cdc.gov/niosh/78127_18.html

Police Scientific Development Branch (1986) *Manual of Fingerprint Development Techniques*, London: Home Office.

Potter, J.A. (1995) *Fatal Justice: Reinvestigating the MacDonald Murders*, New York: W.W. Norton & Company.

Robertson, J. (1992) in *Forensic Examination of Fibres*, ed. J. Robertson, pp. 41–93. New York: Ellis Horwood.

Saferstein, R. (1981) Criminalistics: An Introduction to Forensic Science, Englewood Cliffs, NJ: Prentice Hall, pp. 157–190.

Scientific Working Group for Materials Analysis (SWGMAT) (1998) *Forensic Fiber Examination Guidelines*. Available at http://www.fbi.gov

Smith, R.F. (1990) *Microscopy and Photomicrography: a Working Manual*. Boca Raton, Florida: CRC Press, pp. 1–57.

Tungol, M.W., Bartick, E.G. and Montaser, A. (1991) *Spectochimica Acta Electronica*, 46B, 1535E–1544E.

CHAPTER 3

TRACE EVIDENCE AS INVESTIGATIVE LEAD VALUE

Amy Michaud

INTRODUCTION

The concept of two objects coming into contact with one another and exchanging material is a simple one to grasp. Just picture someone sitting in a freshly painted chair and the idea of how one material can be transferred to another after contact becomes obvious. Locard's brilliant revelation was that there is always an exchange of material after contact, but many times the material is too small to be seen or detected.

Locard's Exchange Principle lays the foundation for why trace evidence examinations are performed, and also why they are so important. On some microscopic level, trace evidence is almost always left behind, or removed from, the scene of a crime. This exchange of minute material even occurs when measures are taken by the suspect to limit the amount of material transferred. A suspect can wear gloves to conceal his or her fingerprints; wear a condom to try to avoid leaving DNA evidence; or throw away their shoes to eliminate the possibility of footwear evidence. The power of trace evidence lies in the fact that, even when taking great care, it is virtually impossible to keep extremely small or microscopic items such as hairs and fibers from being transferred.

Once trace materials are transferred, they can often be compared to known items from the suspect(s), victim(s), or crime scene(s), to help reveal an association. A comparison of this type often requires that the authorities have a suspect identified first. Unfortunately, in the early part of an investigation, the identity of the perpetrator is not always known. In this case, trace evidence may also be used to provide valuable information that could assist investigators in locating the person, or persons, responsible for the crime.

THE CRIMES

During a four-year period from 1988 to 1991, a series of similar sexual assaults took place in several areas of Michigan and Northwest Ohio. Eight victims, both male and female, ranging in age from seven to eighteen, were eventually identified and linked to the same suspect by the similarities of each crime, and by the trace evidence that was ultimately recovered. In every case, the victims were either riding bicycles or walking along rural roads, when they noticed a man drive by them several times. The man would eventually approach the youths, pretending to need assistance, and then get them into his car by threatening them with a blue steel .38-caliber revolver. He was normally wearing something to hide his identity, such as a hat, sunglasses, or mask, when he approached his victims, saying "Get into the car, and don't look at me!". Once inside the vehicle, the kidnapper would tell the victims to get down onto the floor in front of the passenger-side front seat. He would then give the victims a piece of duct tape and have them place it over their own eyes. After that, the suspect would throw what was described as "a blue blanket with a zipper" or a coat, over the top of them to further obscure their view and hide them from any passing vehicles. The attacker would then normally drive some distance making a number of turns, possibly to be sure that the victim would not be able to find the same location again. While driving, the suspect would order the victims to remove their clothing. Subsequent interviews with each of the victims revealed that once their clothes were removed, the suspect would take the garments and place them somewhere in the back of the vehicle. It was believed that the suspect might have placed the clothing in a bag, or onto a tarp of some kind, in order to limit the transfer of trace evidence. Once they reached a secluded area, the suspect would often have the victims get out of the car, and then he would bind their hands with a cord or duct tape. The man would often whip the victims with what was believed to be his belt, telling them that if they didn't do as he wished, he would beat them again. He would then order them to perform oral sex on him. Each victim was eventually driven to a location where they were set free, but only after the suspect took back the duct tape and bindings, and instructed them to collect all of their personal belongings from his car. He even told some of the victims that he didn't want them "leaving any evidence behind".

Several victims were abducted in different areas of the state before authorities realized that the same person might be responsible for the sexual assaults. The similarity of the crimes finally prompted the local law enforcement to form a task force made up of seven different police agencies. The task force collected descriptions of the suspect, and of the vehicle, from all of the possible victims. The attacker was identified as a white male of medium height, with brown hair. His vehicle was described as being white, with a blue interior, bucket seats, and a manual transmission. Although no physical evidence had been collected on the few established cases at that point, the task force decided that if any future victims were identified, the collection of physical evidence would be a primary concern. They also decided that it would be beneficial to send all evidence collected in the future through one central laboratory for examination.

ANALYSIS

The crime laboratory first became involved in this investigation when a fifteen-year-old boy was kidnapped while riding his bicycle home from school. The victim was stopped by a man driving a white car, and forced into the vehicle at gunpoint. The victim's head was covered; and he was driven around for several hours before he was taken to a secluded place and sexually assaulted. After the attack, the suspect drove the youth to an area in the country where he could see a house in the distance. The victim was taken to the center of the road and faced towards the house, while his attacker stood close behind him. The man removed the bindings that held his wrists, and the tape that covered his eyes. He then told the boy "Don't look back, just run to the house and don't look back." Once the boy reached the house, he called his mother. The local Sheriff's Department, who had already been contacted about his disappearance, was alerted.

Task force members immediately recognized similarities between this attack and the earlier abductions that they had been investigating. The victim's clothes were promptly collected and submitted to the laboratory for examination. Upon arrival at the laboratory, the clothes were sent to the Trace Evidence Unit, where they were scraped down and tape lifted in an effort to collect any trace materials that might be present. The clothing items were then turned over to the Biology Unit, where they were inspected for the presence of any biological fluids or hairs. A sexual assault kit was also collected and examined for foreign hairs, fibers, or biological fluids. No unidentified biological stains or human hairs unlike the victim's were found on any of the submitted items.

An examination of the tape lifts and debris removed from the victim's clothing revealed an abundance of animal hairs and blue carpet type fibers. These animal hairs and fibers were mounted on glass microscope slides for further examination and identification. The hairs were examined using a compound microscope, and identified as cat hairs by their general morphology (Figure 3.1a–b). The victim's family owned two cats, so known hair samples were obtained from them. These samples were collected so that they could be used for comparison or elimination purposes if a suspect was eventually apprehended.

The blue fibers that were removed from the victim's clothes were examined using a polarized light microscope (PLM). The optical properties of these fibers were observed, and they were identified as being polypropylene type fibers with a round cross-section and a dull luster (Figure 3.2). The identification of the fiber type was confirmed by the use of a Fourier Transform Infrared Spectrophotometer (FTIR), which also identified the chemical structure of the polymer used to make up the fibers as polypropylene. Polypropylene fibers like

Figure 3.1
*Cat hairs found on
clothing of victim.*

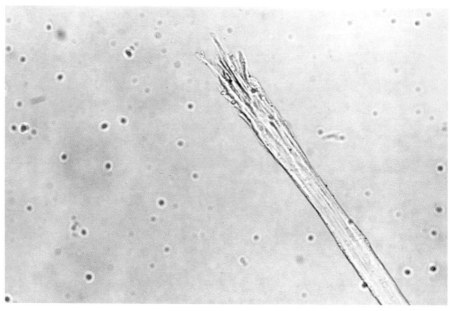

(a)

(b)

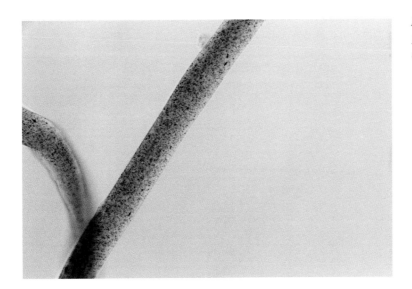

Figure 3.2
Polypropylene fibers found on clothing of victim.

the ones found on the victim's clothes are commonly used to make up floor mats, as well as the carpet found on the doors, back of seats, and rear cargo areas of many vehicles. This finding helped corroborate the victim's statements regarding the interior color of the suspect's vehicle.

Approximately two months after the previous attack, the suspect picked up another victim. A nineteen-year-old female was abducted from a rural area of southern Michigan and sexually assaulted in a similar fashion to the others. While canvassing the neighborhood near where the abduction took place, investigators interviewed someone who saw a white vehicle in the area. The witness stated that the vehicle he saw was an Oldsmobile.

The task force quickly gathered the victim's clothing, along with a sexual assault kit, and sent it to the laboratory for examination. In this case, the victim stated that the suspect had her take off all of her clothes and placed them out of the way, with the exception of her socks. Again, the clothes were sent to the Trace Evidence Unit to be scraped down and tape lifted before sending them to the Biology Unit for further examination.

The Biology Unit examined the victim's clothing for the presence of any biological fluids or hairs. Chemical and microscopical examination of the victim's panties confirmed the presence of spermatozoa; however the victim claimed that she was forced to perform oral sex on the suspect, and that she was not ever vaginally assaulted by him. Further interviews with the victim revealed that she had sexual relations with her boyfriend a short time prior to the attack; therefore, finding biological fluids on the victim's panties was inconsequential in this case. No human hairs dissimilar to the victim's were found on any of her clothing.

Figure 3.3
Polypropylene fibers found on clothing of second victim.

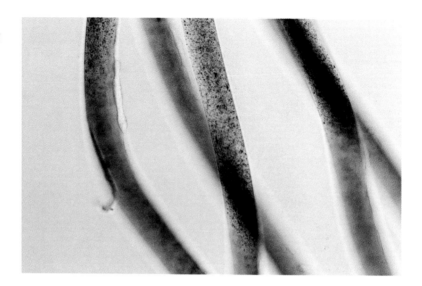

The Trace Evidence Unit examined the tape lifts and debris from the victim's clothing for anything of possible evidential value. The lifts and debris from the socks contained numerous carpet type fibers, while the remainder of her clothes revealed relatively little known trace evidence except for a few animal hairs that were not suitable for comparison purposes.

Four distinct types of carpet fibers were found on the victim's socks. Blue polypropylene fibers with a round cross-section and a dull luster were identified with the polarized light microscope and further confirmed using the FTIR. These fibers were compared to the blue polypropylene fibers found on the previous victim, and determined to be consistent in microscopic properties (Figure 3.3). This finding helped to establish that the two victims could have been in contact with the same object shortly before their clothes were collected. Since the clothing was obtained just after the abductions, the presence of similar polypropylene fibers helped to confirm that the same individual might have been responsible for both crimes.

The three remaining carpet fiber types found in abundance on the victim's socks were determined to be medium blue trilobal nylon fibers with a bright luster, dark blue trilobal nylon fibers with a dull luster, and gray trilobal nylon fibers with a dull luster (Figure 3.4a–c). Since the witness claimed that he saw an Oldsmobile near the scene, General Motors (GM) was contacted in an effort to determine if these fibers may have come out of one of their vehicles. General Motors master standards were obtained through the company, and were compared to the nylon fibers found on the victim using a comparison micro-scope. None of the master standards matched all of the questioned nylon fibers exactly, however the color and appearance of some of the nylons from the

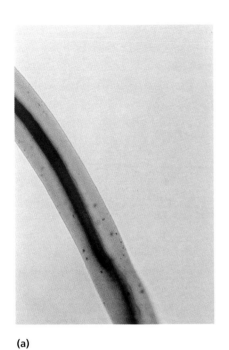

(a)

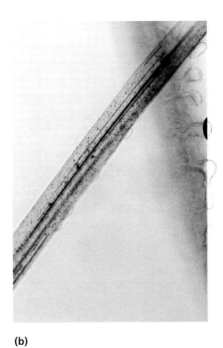

(b)

Figure 3.4
Three different fibers
found on clothing of
second victim.

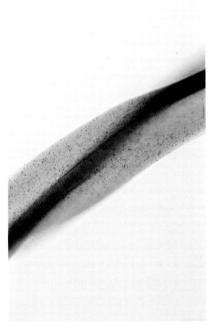

(c)

victim's socks were consistent to certain fibers from a standard named "Deep Sapphire Blue". This carpet was made up of yarns called "12-oz. Trianon". An engineer who worked for General Motors was contacted, and he determined that a company by the name of JPS Automotive Products Corporation made this particular carpet for use in a number of GM vehicles.

JPS Automotive was contacted, and they provided additional information about the carpet in question. "Trianon" was a name GM assigned to fabrics tufted with a 2.25:1 blend of 100 per cent nylon yarn. The fibers used to produce the "Trianon" blends changed several times during the carpet's production, which would account for the GM standard not matching the questioned fibers exactly. They did confirm, however, that each manufacturer uses slightly different colors in their vehicles. The fact that the color of the questioned fibers matched the GM standard helped to confirm the witness's account that he did see a General Motors vehicle. Further information from the company revealed that this carpet was used in several General Motors vehicles in the late 1980s, and specifically with regard to Oldsmobiles it was used in the Toronado, Cutlass, Olds 88, and Calais.

General Motors was contacted with this new information, and they provided a list of people owning vehicles of this type in Michigan and Ohio; however, the list was too large to be of any real value.

While Detectives in Michigan were continuing their investigations, authorities working for the New York State Police were investigating the homicide of a young boy. During their investigation, they heard about the task force that had been formed in Michigan. Some of the circumstances surrounding the homicide in New York and the sexual assaults in Michigan were similar. The New York State Police made arrangements to bring the trace evidence from their homicide case to Michigan. They requested that it be compared to the trace evidence found on the sexual assault victims in an attempt to determine if there was a connection between the cases.

Examination of the trace evidence from the homicide in New York revealed three different types of blue nylon carpet fibers, as well as blue polypropylene fibers. These were compared to the fibers found on the victims in Michigan with the use of a comparison microscope. The blue polypropylene fibers from the homicide victim were compared to the blue polypropylene fibers from the previous two sexual assault cases. Although the fibers were consistent in fiber type, the polypropylene fibers found on the homicide victim had a bright luster, while the polypropylene fibers from the sexual assault victims in Michigan had a dull luster. Further comparison of the three different types of nylon carpet fibers from the homicide victim to the three types of nylon carpet fibers found on the socks of the victim from the most recent sexual assault showed slight dissimilarities in color and physical appearance. The remainder of the trace evidence was also compared but no connection could be made between the homicide in New York and the sexual assaults in Michigan. This elimination convinced investigators in New York that there was no connection between their homicide and the crimes in Michigan, which allowed them to focus their efforts on other, potentially more viable suspects.

The task force continued to develop a number of suspects during this time period. Many investigators felt that the person responsible for these crimes may be involved with law enforcement, since they seemed to have some knowledge of physical evidence. The investigation even focused on a retired police officer for a short period of time, however no evidence ever pointed to him as a likely suspect. The identification of the vehicle soon became the primary concern for the task force.

Approximately one month after the previous incident, a thirteen-year-old female in Northern Ohio was abducted and sexually assaulted. The circumstances surrounding the crime made it immediately apparent that the same suspect was responsible. During this incident, the victim was able to see below the tape that she was forced to place over her own eyes. She was able to describe the interior of the vehicle a bit better, and noticed that the emergency brake between the two front seats had a herringbone pattern on it.

General Motors was contacted once again and given the information about the emergency brake. They were able to determine that a herringbone pattern of this type had been used on a number of their vehicles over the years; however of the four vehicle types previously identified by the carpet fibers, only the Oldsmobile Calais used this type of emergency brake. They were also able to determine that this brake style was used only from 1986 to 1988 (Figure 3.5).

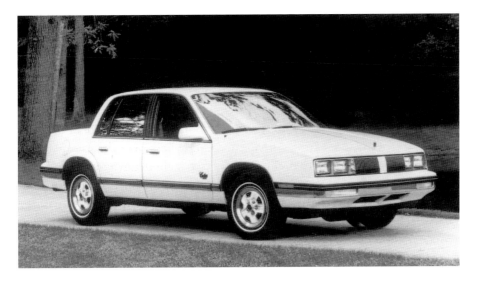

Figure 3.5
Oldsmobile Calais similar to the one driven by the suspect.

Given this information, General Motors provided authorities with a list of all 1986 to 1988 Oldsmobile Calais in Michigan and Ohio that were white with a five-speed manual transmission. Nineteen vehicles were identified, and of those vehicles, only six had a blue interior.

Investigators immediately started background checks on the owners of the six vehicles matching the victim's descriptions. One of the individuals on the list stood out immediately, since he was investigated in 1974 for allegedly kidnapping a young female and driving her around while she was covered with a blanket. The victim in that case was not sexually assaulted, and chose not to prosecute. A photograph of the suspect taken at the time of that incident in 1974 was compared to a composite made from the recent victim's descriptions and found to be similar. Further investigation of the possible suspect revealed that he was a 49-year-old businessman with a wife and a 12-year-old son. Aside from the alleged kidnapping, his criminal record showed that he had been convicted of assault and battery in 1978. Other records revealed that he owned a .38-caliber five-shot revolver, and he needed corrective lenses to drive. Two of the victims had said that the suspect was wearing glasses when he confronted them.

Given this information, investigators started surveillance on the potential suspect. They also started proceedings to obtain known carpet samples from the other five vehicles that were provided on the list from General Motors.

Carpet samples were gathered from the five Calais on the list that did not belong to the potential suspect. These samples were sent to the crime laboratories in Michigan and Ohio for comparison to questioned fibers found on the last three victims. The known carpet samples from the five vehicles were mounted on glass microscope slides and compared to the questioned carpet fibers found on the victims using a comparison microscope. None of the fibers found on the victims were similar in microscopic properties to any of the known carpet samples from the five Oldsmobile Calais. The fact that the fibers from those cars did not match any fibers found on the victims quickly eliminated the owners of those vehicles as potential suspects.

The primary suspect was then put under surveillance for approximately one month. He was observed on numerous occasions driving his Calais for hours, often circling around the same neighborhood for extended periods of time. He was also seen a number of times driving around the local elementary and junior high schools. It was common for him to apply the brakes or even stop his vehicle when passing by children, even when there were no stop or yield signs present, and when the children were not near enough to the street for him to be concerned about their safety. The suspect was also known to turn the vehicle around and pass by some of the children a second time.

The suspect was never seen forcing anyone into his vehicle during the time he was under surveillance; however authorities felt that his driving activity, along with the prior accusation of an abduction, vehicle information, and suspect description was enough to obtain a search warrant for his vehicle and residence.

The suspect's vehicle was brought to the laboratory garage and processed for anything that might have some evidential value. A number of items were collected, including known carpet samples from the floor, door panels, and trunk. The floor mats were collected, and the floors were vacuumed for trace evidence. Tape lifts were taken from the seats, and several possible biological stains were cut from the seat fabric. Known samples of the seat fabric were also collected. The vehicle was processed for latent prints using super-glue fuming and various traditional and fluorescent latent fingerprint powders, along with an alternate light source. A number of latent lifts were obtained using these methods.

The suspect's residence was subsequently searched and a number of items were collected including a .38-caliber Charter Arms five-shot revolver with a blue finish. Two blue blankets were collected as well as a number of baseball hats, white rope or cord, a roll of duct tape, various papers and receipts, and two Michigan county maps. The suspect had two cats at his residence, so known hairs were obtained from both of them as well.

Items removed from the suspect's vehicle and residence were initially compared to the evidence found on the two most recent victims from Michigan, since no physical evidence had been collected after any of the previous attacks. All of the items collected from the vehicle and residence would then be turned over to the laboratory in Ohio for comparison to any evidence that they may have obtained from the abductions that took place there.

The blue polypropylene fibers found on the clothing of both Michigan victims were compared to known fibers from the suspect's Oldsmobile Calais using a comparison microscope and FTIR. The fibers that were used to make the floor mats from the vehicle were determined to be blue polypropylene fibers with a round cross-section and a dull luster (Figure 3.6). These fibers were found to be consistent in microscopic properties to the fibers found on the victim's clothes. The fact that the fibers found on the victim's clothes could have come from the floor mats in the suspect's vehicle gave investigators the first piece of physical evidence to link a suspect to these crimes.

Upon examination of the floor mats, it was noticed that a manufacturers name of "Pretty Products Industries", as well as a serial number, mold number, and date code were all listed on the back. The company was contacted, and they stated that those particular floor mats were only sold in retail outlets, and were never used as original equipment in any vehicles. The company also stated that the date code on the mats indicated that they were produced in 1986. They

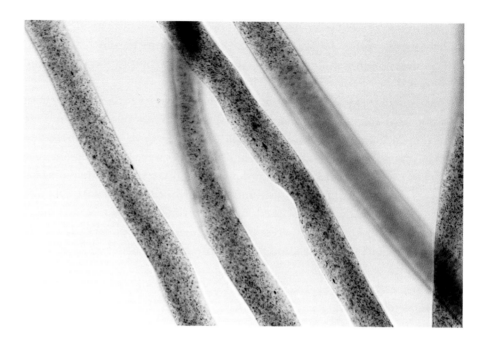

claimed that the fiber content did change from time to time depending on suppliers, however they could not estimate how many mats were made using those same blue polypropylene fibers. Due to the fact that the floor mats were distributed to a relatively large area, and because at least five years had passed since they were produced, it could not be determined how many mats of this type were still being used by the general public in Michigan and Ohio.

Trace evidence examinations continued with the comparison of animal hairs. The suitable cat hairs found on the young male victim's clothing were compared to the known cat hairs from both of his own cats, as well as to the known hair samples from the two cats owned by the suspect. The hairs were compared to each other by mounting them on glass microscope slides, and then viewing them side by side with the use of a comparison microscope.

A majority of the animal hairs found on the victim's clothes were determined to be microscopically similar to the known hair from his own cats. Several of the hairs obtained from the victim's clothes, however, were determined to be consistent in microscopic characteristics to the known hair from one of the suspect's cats (Figures 3.7a and b). Those hairs could not be positively identified back to that cat, since hair evidence, particularly animals', is not an absolute means of identification; however it may be stated that they could have come from the suspect's cat. Although the victim never came in direct contact with the suspect's cat, the hairs could have been transferred indirectly to the victim's clothes, via the car seat or suspect's clothing. This type of indirect transfer could have easily occurred, since numerous cat hairs were obtained from the tape lifts

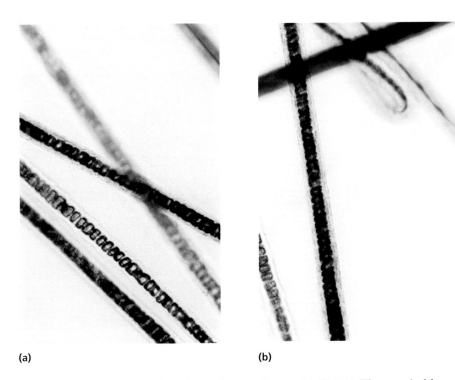

Figure 3.7
Cat hair from (a) clothing
of first victim and (b) the
suspect's vehicle.

(a)   (b)

and vacuum sweepings taken from the interior of the Calais. Those suitable cat hairs from the vehicle were examined, and all of them were determined to be microscopically consistent to the hair from the suspect's own cats.

The known floor carpet samples from the Calais were then examined microscopically and found to consist of medium blue trilobal nylon fibers with a bright luster, dark blue trilobal nylon fibers with a dull luster, and gray trilobal nylon fibers with a dull luster (Figures 3.8a–c). These were compared to the three different types of nylon carpet fibers found on the young female victim's socks. All three of the fiber types that made up the carpet of the suspect's vehicle were found to be consistent in microscopic properties to those found on the victim. The fibers found on the victim's socks could have come from the carpeting of the Oldsmobile Calais owned by the suspect.

The tape lifts and scrapings from both victims' clothing, along with the tape lifts and vacuum sweepings from the suspect's vehicle, were re-examined to determine if any similar trace items were present between the samples from the victims, and the samples obtained from the suspect's car or home.

A number of blue acrylic fibers with a round cross-section and a dull luster were found on the young male victim's shirt. Fibers that were microscopically consistent to these were also found on the tape lifts from the front passenger seat of the Calais (Figures 3.9a and b). The blankets from the suspect's residence were examined in an effort to determine the source of these fibers, but none of the blanket fibers were found in the car or on either victim. No

Figure 3.8
Three types of nylon fibers that make up the carpet of the suspect's vehicle.

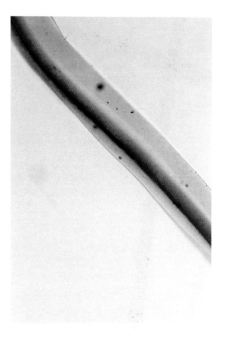

(a)

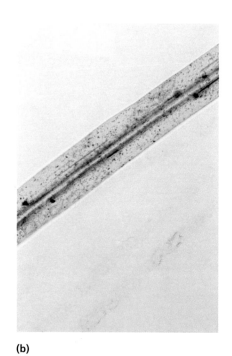

(b)

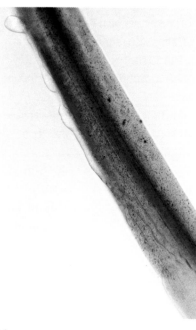

(c)

(a)

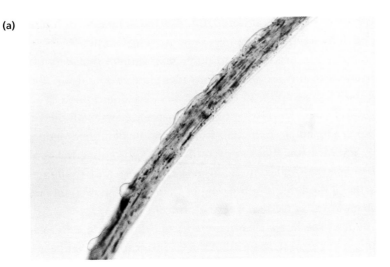

Figure 3.9

Questioned acrylic fibers from (a) clothing of first victim and (b) the suspect's vehicle.

(b)

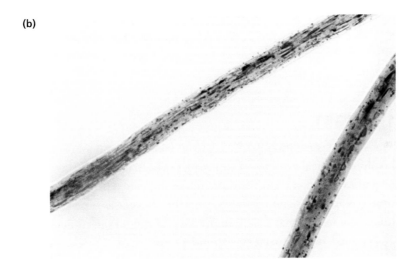

known source for the blue acrylic fibers could ever be determined, however their presence on both the victim's shirt and in the suspect's vehicle strengthened the association between the two.

Blue printed cotton fibers were found in abundance on the tape lifts of both the driver's and passenger's side seats from the vehicle. Printed blue cotton fibers of this type were also found on the tape lifts from the female victim's T-shirt. No known source for these fibers could ever be located either. It was speculated that different blankets or items may have been used to cover each child, and that after the assaults, the suspect disposed of them.

Once the trace evidence was examined, all of the collected evidence items were forwarded to the Biology Unit for examination. Numerous human head hairs and over one hundred and fifty pubic hairs were found on the tape lifts and in the vacuum sweepings from the vehicle. These hairs were examined and compared to head hair and pubic hair samples that were eventually obtained from all of the previous victims identified in Michigan, and to the suspect's known hair samples. Most of the hairs were determined to be consistent to the suspect's own hair. None of the remaining hairs from the vehicle were microscopically similar to the hair from any of the identified victims.

Several stains that were found in the Oldsmobile Calais and on one of the blankets removed from the suspect's residence were examined and identified as seminal fluid. Secretion typing of these stains showed blood group substances that were all consistent with the suspect.

All of the latent lifts obtained from the vehicle were compared to known inked fingerprints from all of the victims, and to the suspect. All of the identifiable prints that were recovered from the car were determined to have been made by the suspect.

The suspect was placed in a personal line-up, and all eight victims were given a chance to identify the person who assaulted them. Two of the victims were able to identify him by sight, and another three identified him as their attacker by hearing his voice.

SUMMARY

The suspect was ultimately brought to trial in Michigan on the two cases that involved physical evidence. Prosecutors in both cases felt that the trace evidence testimony was crucial to the outcome of the trial. For this reason, considerable time was spent educating the jury on the transfer and persistence of hairs and fibers. A court display was then used to aid the jury in understanding the fiber and animal hair associations found in each case. Finally, the significance of these findings was discussed at length, so that the jury could determine the weight to give the evidence.

The suspect was found guilty and sentenced to 20 to 30 years for first-degree criminal sexual conduct, 10 to 15 years for second-degree criminal sexual conduct, 20 to 30 years for kidnapping, and a mandatory two years for committing a felony with the use of a firearm. All of the sentences were to be served consecutively.

The case was discussed with some of the jurors after one of the trials, and they claimed that it was the trace evidence that proved significant to their verdict. Furthermore, the jurors directly attributed the fiber and hair evidence as the crucial factors in their decision.

This case clearly shows the significance of trace evidence by helping to prove that there was an association between the victims and the suspect. This case also demonstrates two other key aspects of trace evidence that increase its potential significance with regard to criminal cases.

The first important aspect revolves around the fact that a suspect can rarely keep all trace material from being transferred, even when they are aware of its value, and even when they take measures to avoid these transfers.

While searching the suspect's home in this case, investigators noticed that the suspect had a number of books in his library dealing with the subject of physical evidence. Subsequent interviews with the suspect revealed him to be a very intelligent man, who seemed to know a lot about the different types of evidence, and about what can be determined through laboratory examinations. This awareness that he had of evidence and its value may have been the reason that a relatively small amount of physical evidence was left behind.

The suspect in this case appeared to do everything in his power to limit the amount of evidence that could be collected. He hid his identity to the best of his ability by wearing a hat and glasses, and then he covered the victim's eyes as quickly as possible so that they could not provide a good description of him to the authorities. The suspect may have even worn the hat to limit the transfer of his hair to the victims. The piece of duct tape that he gave each victim to cover his or her eyes with was always previously cut from the roll. It was speculated that he did this because he didn't want them handling the roll of tape and leaving fingerprints. He always collected, and apparently disposed of the tape, and any ropes or cords used to bind the victims' hands, which effectively eliminated any chance of them being compared or physically matched to anything in his possession. The suspect also drove the victims around for a long time, making many turns and stops on the way to the area where he would assault them, and then he would do the same thing on the way back. The whole journey was made with their eyes and head covered, which made it impossible to return to the area where the assault took place and gather any evidence that may be there. No blanket or coat used to cover each victim was ever recovered, and it was possible that a new one was used each time and then disposed of to eliminate the chance of trace evidence being found. The victim's clothing was always removed and placed out of the way, perhaps to limit fiber and hair transfers. This was probably also done to eliminate the chance of depositing any biological fluids on them during the assaults, which always took place outside of the vehicle. None of the victims were ever vaginally or anally assaulted, so again, recovery of biological fluids would be difficult if not impossible. Finally, the victims were always let out on a paved road, even when most of the roads they traveled on during the kidnapping were gravel. It was believed that this may have been done to cut down on the chance of any tire tracks being left behind.

The suspect in this case had an obvious awareness of the value of evidence. He took great care to avoid leaving anything of evidential value behind, yet trace evidence can be so small that it is impossible to always keep it from being transferred.

Criminals today are becoming more and more educated about the power of physical evidence by watching movies and reading books dealing with the subject. Television programs devoted entirely to forensic science are being shown daily, and high-profile criminal cases are being played out in front of the entire nation on a regular basis. The fact is that many criminals are becoming better at what they do because they have been taught how to avoid leaving evidence behind. In the past, it has been common for someone committing a crime to wear gloves, because they have been aware of the value of latent prints for many years. Now, it is common for a suspect to wear a condom while committing a sexual assault and then to take the condom with them in efforts to avoid leaving DNA behind. Suspects are hiding their identities better because of their awareness of security cameras, and they are disguising their handwriting because they know that it can be identifiable. It has become common now for criminals to dispose of their shoes, clothing, and other items used in a crime to keep investigators from linking them to a victim or scene. Suspects have even been known to shave or use depilatories over their entire bodies to stop hairs from being transferred.

In a time when criminals are going to such extremes to avoid leaving evidence behind, trace evidence has become even more valuable than it had been in the past. It is not uncommon for cases to rely completely on trace evidence, since many times nothing else of evidential value is recovered. Unfortunately, when laboratories should be building up their trace evidence units by providing people, training, and equipment, many laboratories are choosing to do away with them completely.

There are a number of reasons why laboratories might be letting their trace units dwindle to extinction. It takes a long time to train a trace examiner because of the wide variety of items they may be called upon to examine. This may include the examination of things like fibers, hairs, glass, paint, tape, soils, explosive residues, and building materials to name a few. Since any type of substance that can be removed from, or left behind at, the scene of a crime can be used as evidence, a variety of more uncommon materials may also be submitted to the laboratory for identification or comparison. Items such as cosmetics, feathers, glitter, leather, and even popcorn salt have been submitted as evidence in casework. It is often up to the trace evidence examiner to perform the analyses on these types of items because of their vast knowledge of microscopy, chemical methods, and laboratory instrumentation. The time and money necessary to train a trace examiner completely is immense. If a laboratory only has one or two trace examiners, and they retire or leave for some reason, it may be years before a laboratory is able to continue doing trace exams. In a case like this, many labs simply choose to stop examining trace evidence all together.

Another reason some laboratories are getting away from doing trace evidence examinations is because of the many scientific instruments required to do a lot of the analyses. The wide variety of evidence coming into the trace unit requires hundreds of thousands of dollars worth of instrumentation to properly conduct many of the examinations, and some laboratories are not willing to pay the cost to keep a trace evidence unit running. Today's laboratories are sinking much of the money they are given into the newer, more "sexy" sciences such as DNA. The financial burden placed on a laboratory is truly incredible. It is imperative, however, that the managers of crime laboratories and those officials responsible for funding realize the contributions made by every unit in the laboratory. There are many crimes that cannot be solved without the trace evidence examinations, and it is unacceptable for those crimes to go unsolved due to lack of funding and knowledge.

A second important aspect of trace evidence that was highlighted in this case involves the use of trace items to help locate a suspect. Without looking at the fibers and being able to narrow down the list of possible vehicles to a few makes and models, it may have taken much longer to locate a suspect in this case. In fact, it is possible that a suspect may never have been apprehended without the information provided by the fiber examinations.

It is very common for the trace evidence examiner to be given evidence in a case that has hit a dead end, and be asked to give the investigator "any information they can". It is also common for the trace examiner to be able to provide helpful information in a situation like this.

The exchange of materials that constantly takes place when two items come into contact with one another means that an examination of the microscopic particles found on an item can give important clues about the environment(s) that the item has been exposed to. Sometimes this information may be useful because it is distinctive of a particular item or location, as in the previous case. The fibers, along with victim's descriptions, proved to be unique to a particular make of vehicle.

An example of another case which used different forms of trace evidence to identify a specific vehicle, and therefore locate a suspect, involved a hit-and-run which resulted in the death of a twelve-year-old boy. The victim's clothes were brought into the laboratory and examined for trace evidence. Dark maroon and light maroon paint chips were found on the clothing. These were compared to automotive color standards, and it was determined that these colors were used on only a few vehicles in the late 1980s. Laminated glass fragments, consistent with windshield glass, were also found in the victim's clothing. With this information, investigators alerted glass repair shops in the state to inform them if any two-toned maroon, late 1980s vehicles of those few makes and models came in for repairs. One week later, a shop owner called the authorities reporting that a vehicle matching the description had been brought in to have a windshield replaced. A search warrant was obtained, and blood consistent to the victim's, along with hair fragments and fibers consistent to the victim's known hair and clothing were found on the vehicle. The owner of the vehicle was eventually found guilty of the hit-and-run.

Very often the trace materials that are found on items of evidence are not unique enough in themselves to provide useful information to locate a suspect. Finding an orange paint chip on a homicide victim's clothing without knowing its source is not often very useful, just as finding a Negroid pubic hair would only eliminate a small portion of the population. However, a combination of several different types of trace evidence may provide information that can be useful in developing a suspect.

These cases are just a few examples of how trace evidence may be used to help investigators focus in on a suspect. The "lead value" that can be provided by the different forms of trace evidence can be extremely powerful, and is often solely responsible for the eventual capture of a suspect.

CHAPTER 4

PLASTICS IN AUTOMOBILES

Brad Putnam

INTRODUCTION

Physical evidence may take the form of a variety of materials. Most people think of evidence like blood, guns, bullets, and knives when asked what evidence might be present at a crime scene. Perhaps other materials, like hairs or fibers, might be mentioned especially with the advent of modern television shows focusing on forensic science. For law enforcement personnel, recognition of what material is evidence of a crime usually comes from the training and experience of an investigator or forensic scientist.

Unfortunately, many types of physical evidence may be overlooked for a variety of reasons. One of these reasons is a lack of awareness of the significance of a particular type of evidence. This chapter is designed to increase awareness of plastic and polymer evidence in a criminal investigation, specifically investigations involving automotive accidents.

Engineered plastic materials have been examined in forensic laboratories for years. Questions often asked are: did the plastic bag at the dumpsite come from the roll at the suspect's residence? Did the black streak come from the suspect's bumper? Did the melted polymer on the victim's pants come from the passenger's side or driver's side of the vehicle's dashboard? These questions can be answered simply by comparing the sample to the standard without identifying either. While this may be acceptable, additional information may be gathered by identifying the sample and standard.

Historically, forensic analysis has been comparative in nature. However, recently the science has moved into the identification of material and offering more investigative leads. For this reason it has become important to fully characterize evidence material.

A recent development in plastic and polymer evidence is the potential inclusion of polymeric substrates in the Paint Data Query database maintained and disseminated by the Royal Canadian Mounted Police. This would offer the investigator or forensic scientist additional information regarding the type of vehicle the polymer might have originated from. This information requires the identification of the body panel substrate and further supports the need to fully characterize the polymer evidence.

This chapter is designed to aid the examiner in interpreting the analytical results, identifying the polymer evidence, and ultimately gaining a greater understanding of the strength of the polymer comparison.

THE CRIME SCENE

The small red Toyota four-wheel drive pick-up truck approaches the off-ramp intersection fast, 80 miles per hour or more by some accounts. Though the traffic light is red, no effort is made to slow down. Halfway through the intersection, thick skid marks illustrate panic and lost control. The top-heavy truck loses the battle with stability and begins to roll when it hits the soft gravel shoulder of the roadway. The vehicle rolls, strikes a light pole, then violently rolls again before coming to rest, some 250 feet north of the first signs of distress.

The dust barely settles by the time help arrives. A limp and bloody female lies unconscious face down in the short wet grass 50 feet north of the Toyota truck. A badly injured male is upright, yet staggering, beside the resting vehicle. As police and medical personnel attend to the matters at hand, several facts develop. The injuries to both occupants are extensive, but not life-threatening. Both have been drinking. And finally, each accuses the other of being "in control" of the vehicle at the time of the accident. The officer's report of this incident ends as so many do: "the evidence collected was forwarded to the crime lab in an attempt to determine who was driving at the time of the accident. CASE STATUS: Open pending results from crime lab."

The clear and detailed physical evidence often encountered in these types of investigations was not present. Neither occupant had patterned injuries from the seat belts or steering wheel. There were no cracks in the windshield with blood and/or hair. Small bloodstains were collected from various areas of the interior of the vehicle. However, the interpretation of this type of evidence is problematic in roll-over situations.

The critical evidence in this case was a smear of polymeric material on the blue denim jeans worn by the female occupant and blue cotton fibers fused into the polymeric headliner of the truck near the passenger window. The direction and shape of this deposit indicated the transfer occurred with considerable force and speed during the ejection of the victim after the roof had collapsed.

Attention was now turned to the polymeric material on the left leg, near the knee, of the blue jeans. The first comparison was made to the only polymeric material collected from the vehicle, the headliner. It was determined that the headliner could not be a source for the material on the jeans. After phone conversations with the investigator a subsequent search warrant was issued for the Toyota truck. During the execution of this second warrant considerably more thermoplastic surfaces were collected for examination and comparison.

Material from the glove box, dashboard, right windshield molding, right speaker cover, and right door molding were compared to the polymeric material on the jeans. All of the surfaces were differentiable by FTIR (Fourier transform infrared) spectrometry, and none of them were the source of the material on the jeans. While a source for the smear on the jeans was never identified the extensive sampling allowed the forensic laboratory to exclude a number of possibilities.

ANALYSIS

Polymers, or plastics as they are routinely called, can be defined as a high molecular weight organic compound, natural or synthetic (monomers). A series of monomers is sometimes referred to as a homopolymer. If more than one monomer is used in the same structure, the resulting compound is called a copolymer (Mathias 1984).

Plastics have been around since the late 1800s with the making of celluloid as an imitation for natural products such as ivory or tortoise shell. This was to reduce cost and increase availability. By the 1940s advances in polymer chemistry had transformed plastics from objects of imitation to a preferred substitute that replaced natural material such as steel, glass and wood. Materials like polymethyl methacrylate (acrylic), polyvinyl chloride (PVC) polystryene, polyamide (nylon), and acrylonitrile butadiene styrene (ABS) are among many other polymers generated in the laboratory that have gained acceptance as production material. Today plastic materials are so common that they almost go unnoticed and yet with advancement in molding techniques and experimentation with copolymers and additives, there is still no end to the "plastic age."

Plastics are man-made materials that can be shaped or molded into almost any form and are one of the most useful goods ever created. Plastics can be rigid or rubbery and can be shaped into an endless variety of objects. Engineers have developed plastics that have replaced metal and glass. Automotive manufacturers use these plastics to make products stronger, lighter, longer lasting, easier to maintain and less expensive to make. Automotive makers now commonly use plastic bumpers and fenders in their products and in some cars the entire body is made of plastic. The use of plastic to replace metal parts reduces the overall weight of the vehicle and increases fuel efficiency.

The exterior of the vehicle is not the only location in the automotive industry that plastics are taking over. In the interior plastics are being used to reduce cost, weight, compartment noise and vibration. Plastics are now being manufactured that meet the rigorous demands for safety and visual appearance of the consumer, as well as being cost effective for the manufacture. Some of the new plastic materials can be pre-colored which eliminates the need for painting, and with the addition of certain additives can reduce the susceptibility to scratching or the prominence of a scratch when one occurs.

Using a specific polymer on a vehicle in a particular location depends on a number of things. The visual appearance needed for the location, the amount of sunlight received, the desired feel, along with the cost and availability of the polymer are some of the considerations of an automotive engineer.

Certain polymers, however, are routinely used in various locations of the automobile interior because of their inherent qualities. Urethane foams are commonly used in upholstery cushioning or are covered with a "skin" and used in padded instrument panels, headrests, armrest or a headliner. The instrument panels were traditionally made of several separate components (possibly different polymers) that were held together with a steel rod and painted for visual consistency. Currently the technology allows for integrated instrument panels made of acrylonitrile-butadiene-styrene (ABS), ABS/polycarbonate copolymer, polycarbonate, or polypropylene. The steering wheel is usually made from a pigmented vinyl resin or a pigmented urethane when a soft material is needed.

The forensic significance of plastic and polymers in vehicles has been described by Pabst (1984) and Masakowski *et al.* (1986). During high-speed vehicle accidents the occupants may be forced against plastic parts of the vehicle. This force can create sufficient frictional heat to melt a portion of the plastic part. While the plastic is molten a very stable transfer may occur, fibers from the garment in contact can be deposited on or in the plastic surface or the molten plastic might be transferred to the garment. Once the transfer has occurred and the frictional heat is reduced the plastic will harden again and hold the trace evidence or fabric impression. This type of transfer has been termed "textile-plastic fusing marks" or "fiber-plastic fusions". Fusion evidence indicates high-energy impact between the vehicle occupant and the plastic surface, and the smear on the surface may indicate the direction of travel during the transfer process. This information could assist the investigator in determining the driver of a vehicle.

Fourier transform infrared spectroscopy (FTIR) has been used to characterize plastic materials found in forensic casework. The examiner should consider several things when selecting a methodology for analysis: the amount of sample, whether a technique is destructive or not, and the degree of differentiation or characterization that is needed. FTIR analysis allows for rapid nondestructive characterization of plastic material. As Suzuki (1993) states, there are a number of analytical schemes, sampling techniques and accessories available that expand the analytical capabilities of the FTIR. The use of the microscope attachment on the FTIR for examination of plastic material has become accepted and almost routine, in a number of forensic laboratories (Bartic and

Tungol 1993). Ryland (1995) and Tungol *et al.* (1995) previously have covered the power and ease of the microscope attachment on the FTIR when analyzing paints and fibers. Plastics and polymer are just as easy to sample and the information obtained is just as valuable when analyzed by this method. When a microscope attachment is used the technique only requires extremely small amounts of the polymer, is quick, informative, reproducible and non-destructive. These are desired traits of techniques used in the forensic laboratory.

Use of the microscope attachment in the transmission mode is the most commonly applied method. While working in the transmission mode requires more extensive sample preparation than other methods, it usually generates fewer spectral artifacts. The key point in transmission is sample thickness. The sample needs to be of adequate thickness to obtain decent spectra but not to thick to over-absorb certain regions. This thickness has been described as 2–5 μm (Bartick and Tungol 1993) and can be achieved by cutting a small section of the material and then rolling or pressing it flat. The material should be of uniform thickness to avoid a large amount of scattering that could significantly distort the peak shape and baseline.

The process of flattening the material creates a thin film. This thin film can produce an interference fringe in the IR spectrum, particularly with a "glossy" polymer. While the interference fringe will not interfere with the classification of the polymer, it is unsightly and can hamper the computer's ability to search databases effectively.

After flattening, the sample is placed on a salt or IR window for analysis. If the material has elastic properties, as some polymers do, the examiner should place the material in a diamond anvil cell or another type of compression cell to keep the material a proper thickness.

The above-described method is used for both the questioned sample and the standard material. If the questioned sample was removed from a garment care should be used to avoid fibers or other contaminants being collected along with the polymer in question. Any stray fibers can complicate the interpretation of the FTIR spectra obtained.

If the polymer was not smeared into a thin film during the transfer process, then a thin film of polymer needs to be made, as described previously. If the polymer in question has been scraped off the source, as in the case of a rivet scraping over a polymer surface, the small "powder residue" might be able to be flattened thin enough for analysis without manipulating the sample further.

Frequently the standard material will have to be shaved into thin peels with a scalpel blade, by holding the scalpel at an oblique angle and lightly dragged it over the surface. This action should result in thin shavings of polymer being removed from the surface, which are then analyzed as described above.

Locating the evidence of fiber plastic fusion while processing a vehicle only takes a keen eye and proper lighting. Oblique lighting, as well as direct light should be used while inspecting the dashboard, instrument panel, door covers, interior plastic trim, steering wheel and speaker grills. The examiner should inspect surfaces for any change in the texture; a handheld magnifying lens may aid this inspection. If a change in the texture is noted or the surface appears abraded or scratched, these areas should be inspected further for fibers or fabric impressions. If these materials are present, evidence should be documented, photographed, and the panel should be collected or the area cut out.

In the laboratory the search for fiber plastic fusion evidence on a garment is no different than examining it for other physical evidence. The garment is placed in a well-lit area of the laboratory and searched thoroughly. Special attention should be given to the lower extremities, or raised portions of the garment, such as rivets that are commonly encountered with casual pants. A plastic transfer smear will generally have a glossy appearance. After documenting the location and appearance of the fusion mark (e.g. the direction of deposit, whether the material is on the surface or in the weave of the garment, etc.) it can be collected for examination. The fusion material should then be physically separated from the substrate with the aid of a stereomicroscope, scalpel, tweezers, and a steady hand.

HIGHLIGHT

Often the forensic cases chronicled in texts or on television end in nice neat packages as they are resolved by the analysis or comparison of a pivotal piece of evidence. Unfortunately this is not always the case in the laboratory. While the smear on the headliner told a story of where and when the female victim was ejected from the vehicle, the source of the polymer fusion was not located.

The laboratory's ability to objectively analyze and effectively compare evidence is dependent on the standards provided. Personnel outside of the laboratory often perform the collection of this standard material and therefore it is paramount that the individuals collecting the standards obtain adequate and representative samples of *all* possible sources.

A number of sources for the polymer fusion mark on the jeans were available in the vehicle, such as the headliner, glove box, speaker covers, dashboard, and steering wheel. It is crucial that the investigator not develop "tunnel vision" by investigating the case from only one perspective. In this case the investigators believed the victim to be in the passenger side of the vehicle. As a result, no standards from the driver's side were collected.

All possible source materials should be collected even when there is no visual difference in the object. In the interior of an automobile this is especially true; for functional reasons, automotive engineers will place chemically different polymers in different parts of the car which may be in close proximity to each other. Yet they attempt to make them visually similar for aesthetic reasons.

The successful analysis and comparison of evidence in a case is dependent upon a number of things. These include the ability to recognize the material as evidence, the knowledge to collect the appropriate standards, the training to effectively analyze the materials, and the experience to evaluate the significance of the evidence in the context of the case.

INTERPRETATION

Qualitative analysis, or identification of a polymeric material, may be achieved by interpreting the FTIR spectrum obtained by analysis. Once the spectrum is obtained, the examiner has several methods for identifying the polymer type: the examiner can search an electronic database on the instrument for spectra similar to the questioned spectrum, the major peaks in the questioned spectrum may be compared to a table listing characteristic absorption peaks of various polymers (see Table 4.1), or with experience the examiner may be able to identify the polymer type by sight alone.

Perhaps the simplest method of interpretation is to evaluate the entire questioned spectrum and compare it to a spectrum of known material from a text or laboratory reference library. However, as with any identification method, this should be performed with caution, because occasionally spectra of different material can appear virtually indistinguishable. This is especially true with

		Table 4.1
Acetal	910, 1100, 1240, 1380,1470	*Major absorption peaks*
Acrylonitrile butadiene Styrene (ABS)	2900 (formation), ~2240, 1600, 1490, 1450, 760, 700	*found in polymer analysis.*
Polyamide	1640, 1560, 1275, intense bands 3300–2800	
Terephthalate (polybutylene or polyethylene)	1720, 730, 1265, 1100, 1020, 1410	
Polycarbonate (PC)	~1770, 1500, 1230, 1195, 1160, 1015	
Polyethylene	1470, 2850–2930, strong band ~720	
Polymethyl methacrylate (acrylic)	1730, 1150, 1190, 1240, 1270, 1450	
Polypropylene	1460, 1375, 2850–2950	
Polyurethane	1700, 1590, 1520, 1220	
Styrene	2900 (formation), 1490,1450, 760, 700	
Polyvinyl acetate	1740, 1240, 1020 (note shape), 1370, 1430	
Polyvinyl chloride	1430, 1250, 690	

spectra of large molecules with minor differences (phthalates) or copolymers where there may be slight variations in the minor components.

One of the difficulties with identifying the basic polymer type is the addition of extenders and additives during the manufacturing process, because this material may add bands to the spectrum or obscure polymer band information. Additives are materials that enhance the basic properties of the final polymer product extenders are materials that are usually added to add bulk to the polymer and thus reduce final cost.

While the use of these materials can complicate the identification process, they may be very useful in the comparison of polymers. The combination of additives and extenders are often specific to the manufacturer, end-use application and the time of processing.

Some of the most probative regions of polymer spectrum are the carbonyl region (1630–1780 cm^{-1}) the nitrile region (2220–2260 cm^{-1}) and the region around 3000 cm^{-1}. Often the examiner will start the interpretation of the spectrum at these regions because they will provide quick information of what polymer types may or may not be present. Once these regions have been evaluated, the examiner can evaluate other regions of the spectrum for more specific information.

Two polymers used extensively in plastics are polyethylene and polypropylene. These plastic products have a variety of end uses including pink lawn flamingos, toilet seats, and are finding increased use in the automotive industry. Polypropylene is often used on vehicle instrument panels, door panels, fascias, headliners and trim. The spectra are easily differentiated from each other (Figures 4.1 and 4.2). Another polymer that is easily differentiated is that of acetal resin. Acetal (a polyoxymethylene resin) was used as a one-piece instrument panel for the 1961 Plymouth Valiant (Meikle, 1995). This polymer has a wide range of end-use applications today including disposable lighters, zipper

Figure 4.1

HMW polyethylene. Note the sharp band at 720 cm^{-1}.

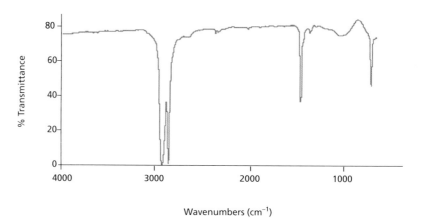

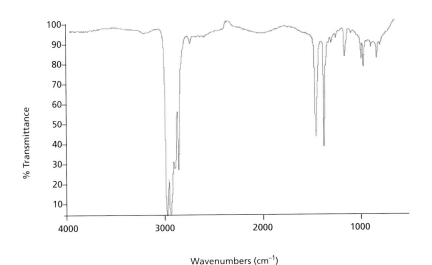

Figure 4.2

Polypropylene. Note the two bands at 1460 cm^{-1} and 1375 cm^{-1} and the absence of the band at 720 cm^{-1}.

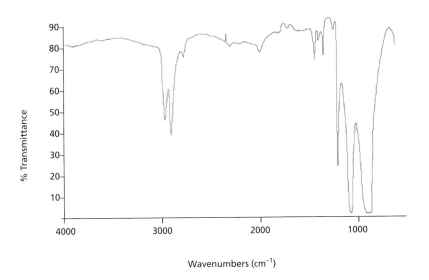

Figure 4.3

Acetal resin homopolymer.

teeth, and interior automobile door handles. The spectrum is very diagnostic with strong absorption bands at 910 cm^{-1} and 1100 cm^{-1} sharp band at 1240 cm^{-1} and no carbonyl peak (around 1730 cm^{-1}) (Figure 4.3).

Nylon (polyamide) is typically thought of as a textile product but has had widespread use as an engineered plastic for over fifty years. The use of polyamide in vehicles is typically in the interior door handles or other ridged support brackets. Another non-textile, non-automotive application that polyamide has seen is in the use of roller-skate wheels. Polyamide's spectrum has strong absorption bands at 2800–3300 cm^{-1} and the amide I and amide II bands at 1640 cm^{-1} and 1540 cm^{-1} are distinctive (Figure 4.4).

Figure 4.4

Polyamide. Note the band formation at 3300–2800 cm^{-1}.

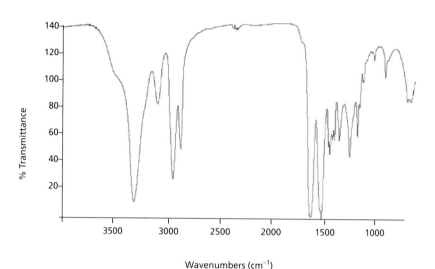

Figure 4.5

Polymethyl methacrylate. Note the strong carbonyl band at 1730 cm^{-1}, and the two doublets around 1190 cm^{-1} and 1270 cm^{-1}.

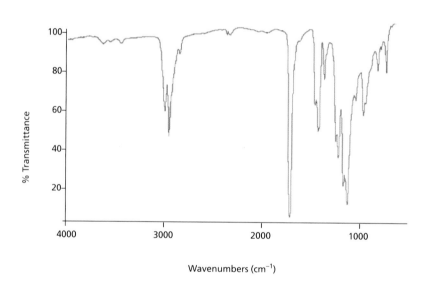

Most acrylics are polymers of methyl methacrylate (PMMA) and have typical end-use application in transparent materials such as lenses, automotive trim, household items, light fixtures and decorator items. The spectrum, as with most homopolymers, is very distinctive for this material (Figure 4.5).

Another engineered plastic that is often used in transparent objects is polycarbonate (PC). Applications for this material are usually those that take advantage of its uniquely high impact strength. However, recent interest in this polymer has been generated due to its low flammability. Currently polycarbonate is being used in reflectors, lenses, headlights, body panels, and mirror housings. The spectral characteristics of this polymer are a strong 1770 cm^{-1},

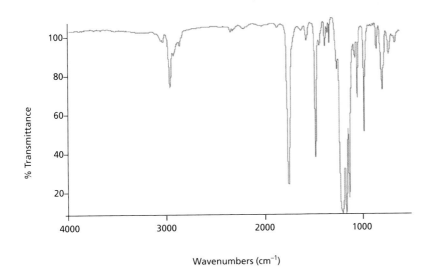

Figure 4.6
Polycarbonate.

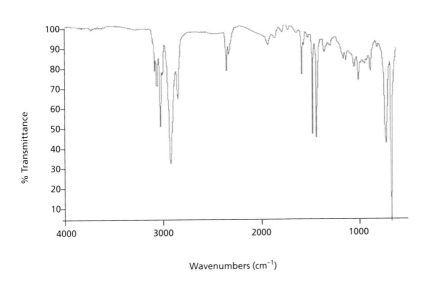

Figure 4.7
Styrene homopolymer.

sharp 1500 cm^{-1} and the unique peaks located at 1230 cm^{-1}, 1195 cm^{-1} and 1160 cm^{-1} (Figure 4.6).

Polystyrene is a clear thermoplastic used in containers, packaging, furniture and other household goods. The spectrum shows "overtone bands" which are small broad peaks located from 2000–1700 cm^{-1}, sharp peaks 1490 and 1450 cm^{-1} and another sharp set of peaks at 760 cm^{-1} and 700 cm^{-1} (Figure 4.7).

Polystyrene's impact strength as a homopolymer is rather low so it is often mixed with other polymers to improve strength or flexibility. Acrylonitrile butadiene styrene (ABS) is a copolymer often found in the interior of automobiles. Released in commercial products in the 1950s, ABS was used in luggage

Figure 4.8

Acrylonitrile butadiene styrene.

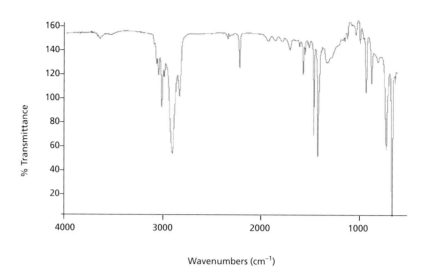

Figure 4.9

Polyurethane Note the strong bands located at 1700 cm^{-1}, 1520 cm^{-1} and 1220 cm^{-1}.

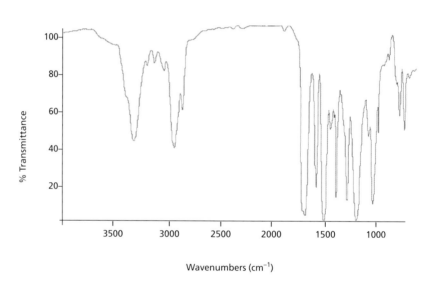

and as one-piece refrigerator trays. Currently, as with many other polymers, ABS is used in a wide variety of applications including the toy industry (Lego®), office accessories, and the console of the new Volkswagen Beetle.

The spectrum of ABS shows the characteristic nitrile band at 2220 cm^{-1}, the small overtone bands at 2000–1700 cm^{-1}, a strong formation around 2900 cm^{-1} and two strong sharp peaks at 700 cm^{-1} and 760 cm^{-1} (Figure 4.8).

Polyurethane usually encountered as "foam" is utilized as insulation to reduce noise and vibration in the automotive industry. The physical appearance of the material, combined with its characteristic spectrum allows a straightforward identification of the material (Figure 4.9).

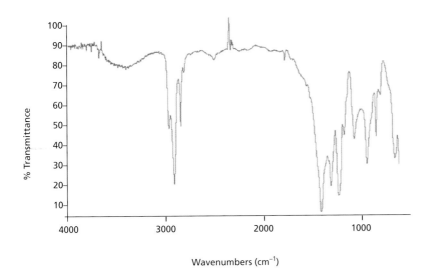

Figure 4.10
Polyvinyl chloride.

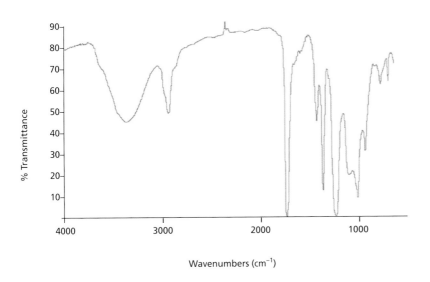

Figure 4.11
Polyvinyl acetate.

The automotive industry will often cover the polyurethane foam with a second material, called a "skin" in the industry. The composition of the "skin" may be a variety of polymers, although polyvinyl chloride (PVC) is routinely used. PVC has a wide range of end-use applications in addition to its use in the automotive industry. Depending on the amount of plasticizers (additives used to increase flexibility), PVC has been found in garden hoses, watch bands, raincoats and wading pools. The spectrum of PVC is readily identified by the prominent bands at 1430 cm^{-1}, 1250 cm^{-1} and 690 cm^{-1}, and the "missing" carbonyl around 1730 cm^{-1}. The examiner will have to exercise caution as the missing carbonyl band may not always be relied on when dealing with PVC.

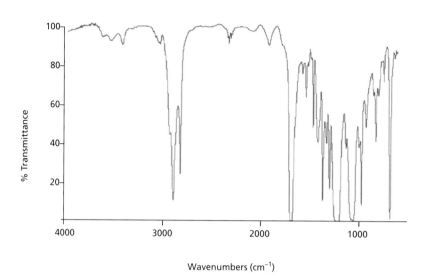

Figure 4.12
Polyethylene terephthalate
(PET).

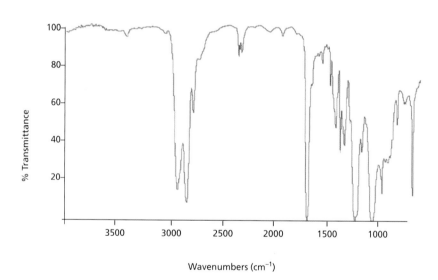

Figure 4.13
Polybutylene terephthalate
(PBT).

Additives may be used to increase stability and flexibility and, depending on the additive, the carbonyl band could be present (Figure 4.10).

Another polyvinyl compound of some forensic significance is polyvinyl acetate (PVA). While not routinely used in the automotive industry PVA is the main compound in some water-soluble glue. Dried PVA on clothing may be confused with a fusion mark, and may be encountered on clothing particularly on children's garments. The spectrum has a unique shape of the bands at 1100 cm^{-1} and 1024 cm^{-1} (Figure 4.11).

Terephthalates as a group are a very popular engineered plastic used in a wide variety of products. In general terephthalates are easily recognized, however the

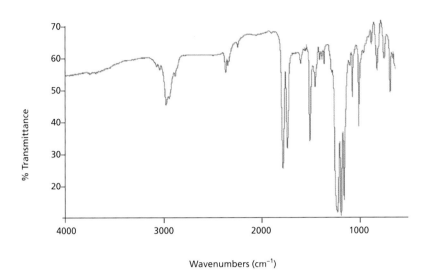

Figure 4.14
Polycarbonate/ABS
copolymer.

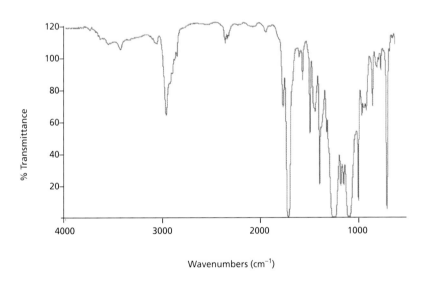

Figure 4.15
Enduran, a PBT/PET
copolymer from GE
plastics.

differentiation between polyethylene terephthalate (PET) (Figure 4.12) and polybutylene terephthalate (PBT) (Figure 4.13) can be quite difficult.

Once the examiner is comfortable recognizing the major absorption bands of the common polymers the identification of copolymers should be fairly direct. This chapter has already covered the identification of a popular copolymer, ABS. Another copolymer that is simple to recognize is a polycarbonate/ABS blend. This spectrum exhibits the polycarbonate peaks already mentioned at 1230 cm⁻¹, 1195 cm⁻¹ and 1165 cm⁻¹, with the additional ABS banding of the nitrile 2220 cm⁻¹ and the styrene sharp peaks at 760 cm⁻¹ and 700 cm⁻¹ (Figure 4.14).

Figure 4.16

Sample from a Toyota dashboard.

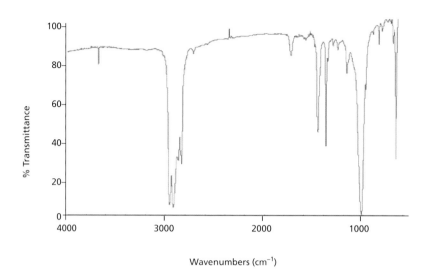

Some copolymers are more difficult to identify. Enduran, for example, is a mixture of polybutylene and polyethylene terephthalate. While as seen earlier the terephthalate is obviously present at 1720 cm⁻¹, 730 cm⁻¹, 1265 cm⁻¹, 1100 cm⁻¹, the interpretation of the smaller bands becomes very important (Figure 4.15).

As with the recognition of copolymers, the more familiar the examiner is with the spectra of the various polymers the easier it is to detect the bands from extenders and additives. Talc, for example is often added to polymers that are used in automotive interior production. Once the polymer "base" is identified the talc peaks are clear. The polypropylene peaks are recognized at 1460 cm⁻¹ and 1375 cm⁻¹, leaving the talc peaks located at 3675 cm⁻¹, 1015 cm⁻¹ and 680 cm⁻¹ (Figure 4.16).

REFERENCES

Bartic, E.G. and Tungol M.W. (1993) "Infrared microscopy and its forensic applications," in *Forensic Science Handbook Vol. III*, ed. R. Saferstein, Regents/Prentice Hall, pp. 196–252.

Masakoski, S., Enz, B., Cothern, J.E., and Row, W.F. (1986) "Fiber-plastic fusions in traffic accident reconstruction," *Journal of Forensic Sciences*, JFSCA, 31(3), July, 903–912.

Mathias, L.J. (1984) "Fundamentals of the polymer chemistry of acrylics and vinyls", *Proceedings of the International Symposium on the Analysis and Identification of Polymers*, Washington DC: US Government Printing Office, pp. 25–38.

Meikle, J.L. (1995) *American Plastic: A Cultural History*, Rutgers University Press.

Pabst, H. (1984) "The textile-plastic fusion mark: Guidepost to the car collision driver," paper presented at the 10th Meeting of the International Association of Forensic Sciences, Oxford, sponsored by the Forensic Science Society, Harrogate, North Yorkshire, England.

Ryland, S. G. (1995) "Infrared microspectroscopy of forensic paint evidence," in *Practical Guide to Infrared Microspectroscopy*, Practical Spectroscopy Series, Vol. 19, ed. H.J. Humecki, New York: Marcel Dekker, Inc., pp. 163–243.

Suzuki, E.M. (1993) "Forensic application of infrared spectroscopy," in *Forensic Science Handbook Vol. III*, ed. R. Saferstein, Regents/Prentice Hall, pp. 71–196.

Tungol, M.W., Bartick, E.G. and Montaser, A. (1995) "Forensic examination of synthetic textile fibers by microscopy infrared spectrometry", in *Practical Guide to Infrared Microspectroscopy*, Practical Spectroscopy Series, Vol. 19, ed. H.J. Humecki, New York: Marcel Dekker, Inc., pp. 245–285.

CHAPTER 5

FINDING TRACE EVIDENCE

Richard E. Bisbing

INTRODUCTION

True crime books and detective fiction are often best sellers and popular television shows tell stories about how detectives search for the perfect method of catching the criminal. Regardless of the way media portrays forensic science, most people recognize that solving a murder, for example, is often a daunting task because in many instances the killers have the advantage of stealth; or, as William Faulker (1991) wrote in 1948, "of all human pursuits, murder has the most deadly need for privacy; how man will go to almost any lengths to preserve the solitude in which he evacuates or makes love, but he will go to any length for that in which he takes life." When a crime occurs in the middle of the night where there are no witnesses, one way to catch the culprit is to find the material evidence left behind. Today, many people think that fingerprints and DNA can solve all crimes and therefore are the perfect methods; but, in fact, they cannot and are not. Trace evidence often must be used instead, including everything from footprints left in the night to traces of dye leached from a new pair of blue jeans. Trace evidence might be anything that can be described as small bits of material, like particles of dust, that are used as associative evidence. These associative materials usually originate from one of the following generic groups: impressions such as from shoes or boots; genetic markers found in blood and semen; samples from the body like hairs; manufactured materials such as fibers, paint, and glass; or soil from the ecological environment. The wise detective will always be looking for evidence from each and every source but, in many cases, it is likely the trace evidence will be invisible, just as the criminals think they are invisible. Therefore, the discovery and recovery of these microtraces often takes special people, a special effort, and special techniques to make them useful to the investigation.

Criminalists know from the principle attributed to the French microscopist Edmond Locard of Lyon that "the microscopic debris that cover our clothes, floors, and bodies are the mute witnesses, sure and faithful, of all our movements and of all our encounters" (Locard 1930). Trace evidence usually fits together like a jigsaw puzzle to paint a picture of what happened and who was the guilty party; but, if detectives are to use trace evidence of all kinds to their best advantage, they should not be limited to what they can see. In the dead of winter, 1980, Saginaw detectives knew they had a difficult case. There was no visible evidence of who killed Ann Presnell[1], so they called the Michigan State Police Laboratory for help.

Early on Saturday, January 5, 1980, a telephone call awakened Sgt. Eugene G. Ambs, a latent print specialist at the Bridgeport Regional Laboratory. The caller was Mark Tennant, a chemist at the laboratory, who just happened to be on call that weekend. Milburn Presnell had returned home to find the partially clad body of his wife, Ann, stabbed and mutilated in their home about two hours after she had left the party they were both attending. The telephone call was the start of a week that would include a 36-hour workday for the forensic scientists and an investigation that pivoted on evidence as small as a single hair, as fragile as a palmprint on wallpaper and as obscure as the impression of one fabric on another. Fresh fallen snow lay on the ground that morning as the crime scene investigators arrived. Soon thereafter, a police spokesman reported that the crime laboratory had apparently found few clues. No one knew early on Saturday morning that valuable clues were still invisible and yet to be discovered.

If forensic science is to be helpful in solving the most difficult of cases, the investigation should start with a well-designed crime scene team, including specialists in each of the disciplines where evidence is likely to be important. Ambs was called because he was part of a five-member unit that identifies finger, palm and foot prints. In other cases, the firearms examiner should be called if there has been a shooting. A rape or violent murder necessitates that the trace evidence examiner and blood spatter specialist is part of the team. It is also best if the team follows a methodical and scientific approach to crime scene investigation, and never relies solely on chance evidence; however, if it comes their way, they need to exploit it to the fullest. The specialist is more likely to recognize the small bit of trace evidence, have the necessary skills to do something with it, and take advantage of the chance happening that will make the case. For the criminal, luck is most important because the unexpected possibility of time or temperature, an object hidden for six days under the snow, or minute particles of which the perpetrator and investigators were unaware will remain after other potential evidentiary materials have been hidden, discarded or destroyed. These chance findings in a case will often prove decisive and someone needs to be there to recognize them.

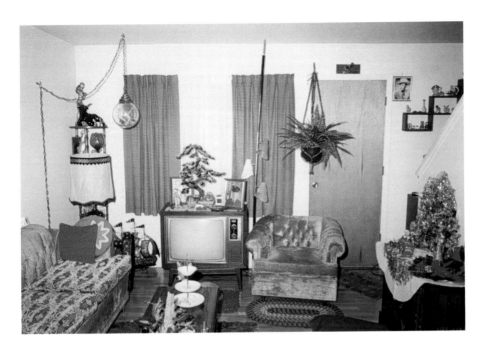

Figure 5.1
Living room in victim's residence looking from the kitchen where the victim's slashed body was found. The landing and stairway leading to the upper floor is in the right rear corner. Latent footwear impressions on the landing showed the killer went up stairs.

THE CRIME SCENE

The crime scene was in a two-storied townhouse, part of an eight-unit building. The first floor included a hallway near the entrance, kitchen, dining area and living room. The furnishings were traditional but inexpensive (Figure 5.1). The home was generally neat and orderly, except for a scatter of underclothing on one of the beds upstairs. The victim was found lying on her back with her head just inside the front door. Her left leg was bent back nearly double at the hip; and her lower leg was partially extended out the front door, holding the outside storm door slightly ajar. She wore a white and blue hospital gown (open back) as a nightgown that covered her upper torso and a green acrylic fleece bathrobe. She had recently been released from the hospital and had been recuperating at home. There were numerous deep lacerations on her face; numerous stab wounds and deep slashes in her chest and upper torso; and deep large gashes in her abdomen, vulva, and both legs. Her head was nearly severed at the neck by knife cuts (Figure 5.2). Some blood was smeared on the floor.

Numerous bloodstains were immediately noted around the front door and several appeared to be bloody fingerprints. Although the latent print specialist carefully photographed each suspected fingerprint impression, it was later determined that none of the bloody fingerprints were identifiable. None of the bloodstains collected at the scene could be shown to be foreign to the victim. No semen was identified either on or in the victim and no semen was detected on any clothing items. It appeared from the outset that fingerprints and blood

Figure 5.2

The victim was found lying on the kitchen floor with her head and shoulders in the entryway. Her left leg propped open the front door. She wore a green fleece bathrobe and white hospital gown.

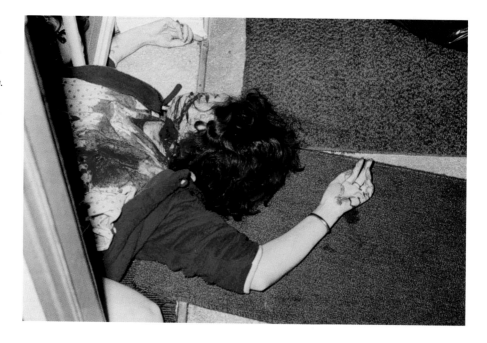

or semen were not going to solve this case. Today, AFIS and DNA data banks are used to locate possible suspects but, in the cold of winter in Saginaw, Michigan 20 years ago, the fingerprints were of no value and DNA was not yet a tool available to the forensic scientists. As the investigators began their search for clues, there was no suspect in sight, and the neighbors had not heard or seen a thing. The case appeared as bleak as the weather.

Crime scene searches start with the most fragile evidence, such as footprints, that could be destroyed just by walking around the crime scene. Footwear impressions may be as positively identifiable as fingerprints because each shoe or boot leaves a unique print and one cannot commit most crimes without moving around the crime scene, thereby leaving footprints. Unfortunately, they are too often neglected. They are more often thought of when searching outdoor scenes than indoors, even though hardwood and tiled floors are very likely to support either prints in previously undisturbed dust or latent prints left in moisture and oils from the shoes or boots.

This case was no different than many others. The investigators had aimlessly milled around, walking on the floors where the killer must have walked earlier. The floors surrounding the body had not been processed for footwear impressions. Although the possibility of detecting footprints where other officers had walked was remote, and the process time-consuming, we dusted the entire kitchen floor, bare hardwood floors in the living room and dining area, stairs to the second floor, and hardwood floors in the upstairs hall and bedrooms. A liberal amount of black powder applied to relatively large pieces of rolled cotton was used in this case as a means to spread powder on floors and walls. This technique works surprisingly well.

Latent footwear impressions were photographed and lifted with transparent tape from the kitchen floor next to the victim's right leg, from the living room floor north of the post containing the foyer closet, and from the landing leading to the upstairs bedrooms. The largest of the three prints was just about four square inches in area. They were only partial prints; and there were two patterns, from two different kinds of soles (Figure 5.3). Whether the two soles were from two perpetrators was not settled until later at a court hearing. In a hallway outside the courtroom, the woman neighbor, who accompanied the husband when he found the body and called the police, was wearing boots that matched the prints from the living room. Only one pattern remained unidentified until the subject's boots were found.

When the suspect's boots were recovered, the latent footwear impressions were compared with inked impressions of the boot soles. Transparencies are often used for comparison and these impressions were amenable to the technique. Some of the inked impressions were made on transparent film and the photographs of the questioned impressions were printed on transparent photographic paper. The impressions can then be overlaid. Sometimes the confusion regarding which impression is being observed (known or questioned) can be alleviated by inserting a white index card between the overlays. When the card is slowly removed, the impressions can be distinguished and carefully compared for individualities.

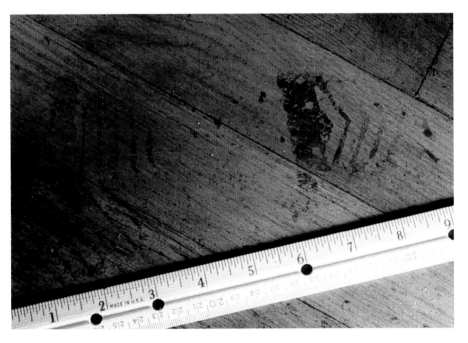

Figure 5.3

Latent footwear impressions were developed on the floor with black fingerprint powder and photographed. This impression was located in the entryway and subsequently identified as belonging to the neighbor who accompanied the husband when the victim was discovered.

Figure 5.4

This footwear impression was located next to the victim's leg on the kitchen floor. It was subsequently identified as being made by the defendant's boot.

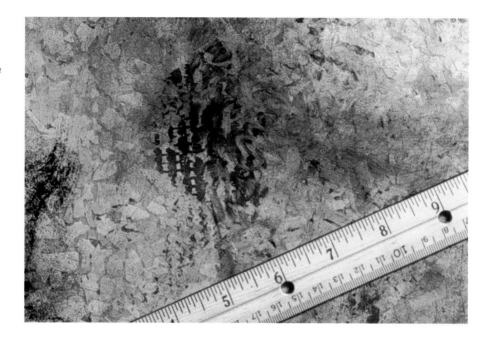

One impression was subsequently identified with boots worn by the woman neighbor. The footwear impression developed on the kitchen floor next to the victim's right leg was identified as having been made by the right brown leather boot recovered from the suspect's residence (Figure 5.4). The footwear impression developed on the landing to the upstairs probably was made by the right brown leather boot recovered from the suspect's residence. All other shoes in the townhouse were eliminated as the source of the footwear impressions on the kitchen floor and landing. No other unidentified impressions were found.

After the footwear impressions were preserved, the victim was searched. Numerous pubic hairs were found on the body. It turned out later that they had been cut with the knife when the victim was slashed. Originally, it was suspected that the killer left them because they were loose on the victim's chest, but later comparison showed they belonged to the victim. While the pubic hairs were being recovered, a blue fabric impression was noted on the white nightgown covering the victim's chest. It appeared as though the color had leached from a new pair of blue jeans. The telltale pattern of a denim-like weave was also visible on the plain weave of the hospital gown.

The walls, refrigerator, stove, table and counter tops in the kitchen were dusted for fingerprints. The victim's arms and legs were dusted with a magna brush for possible prints. Latents were discovered, preserved by photography, lifted with transparent tape, and placed on a transparent plastic backer. Each photograph and tape lift was identified by case number, location, orientation, date and time of collection, and the person lifting the print.

A search of the house produced nothing more of apparent significance and the crime scene was sealed in the event that additional work might be needed following the autopsy and initial police investigation. But crucial evidence had been overlooked.

The nightgown and robe were searched at the laboratory for more microtraces by rolling transparent adhesive tape over the garments and examining the collected debris with a stereomicroscope. At the same time, the comparison of hairs collected from the crime scene was begun using established methods (Bisbing 1982, 2000). These initial efforts were directed to searching for possible foreign hairs in order to provide a lead to the detectives. Sometimes hair color and possible racial origin can be of some help in describing possible suspects to the investigators. Therefore, the questioned hairs were compared with samples taken at the autopsy to determine whether any of the hairs found on the body came from anyone other than the victim. The hairs picked from the body and loose hairs combed from her pubic hair appeared to be hers. They were similar in color, length, diameter, curliness, pigment, surface structure and medulla. The hairs had been cut, apparently during the vulvar slashing.

On the other hand, the lifting tape from the bathrobe revealed one dark brown hair that was triangular in cross section, a characteristic of facial hair, and obviously not the victim's. Foreign hairs and fibers will always be found; how to assess them as evidence is another matter. This was the only foreign hair, a facial hair, recovered from the victim's body, and, at that stage of the investigation, the hair evidence seemed pretty meager. Nevertheless, the facial hair would ultimately take a central role in the investigation and the fact that the victim's pubic hairs were cut would greatly assist with subsequent comparisons.

On Monday, detectives met with the forensic scientists to discuss what they had learned. It seemed that the detectives were pretty much at a loss on how to proceed and were searching for help from the laboratory. Forensic scientists often have to encourage detectives to take advantage of the physical evidence. To keep the interest up, the laboratory team went back to the residence with the detectives to search for footwear in the hopes of eliminating the footwear impressions found because they belonged to the victim or her husband. By Tuesday, everyone associated with the crime scene was satisfied they did not have any shoes that matched the footprints. They must be from the killer. With photographs in hand, the investigators were sent out looking for shoes. If for no other reason, it gives them something to talk about with witnesses and suspects.

On Tuesday, the detectives and forensic scientists went back to the scene again to be certain nothing had been overlooked. The wall over the victim's body was dusted and a palm print was found. Fortunately the house had been

Figure 5.5

The location where the defendant's palm impression was developed on the kitchen wall.

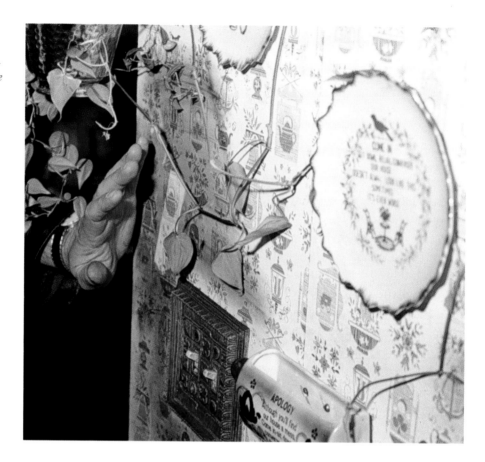

sealed by police to prevent someone from leaving the print on the wall after police first processed the house (Figure 5.5).

As the investigation continued, the detectives brought more fingerprint and palm cards to the laboratory, primarily for elimination. During one of these visits, it became known that Frederico Santiago, who accompanied the victim when she left the party, had a mustache. The detectives now had the last person seen with the victim at the party, a facial hair, a palm print that could not be eliminated, and something to look for, the shoes that left the footwear impressions on the kitchen floor. From that point on, the investigation focused on one person.

The detectives were asked to obtain Santiago's palm and fingerprints and samples of mustache hair. By the time they re-interviewed him, he had shaved his moustache. Although an association was never made between that one facial hair from the bathrobe and known hair from the defendant, it took its place as a linchpin in the solution of the case. Detectives obtained the fingerprints and palm prints, but the palm print from the kitchen wall could still not be identified. Unfortunately, the inked impressions were not taken correctly; the known inked palm impression from Santiago did not record the ridge structure from the hypothenar zone, the heel of the hand.

The detectives asked Santiago whether he would take a polygraph. The investigators were urged to contact him again, and if he agreed, to immediately make the necessary plans for the test before he changed his mind. Santiago agreed to take a polygraph test, which would take place at the laboratory. When he arrived for the polygraph, Santiago was asked for another set of prints. He agreed.

Three rooms away, preparations were made to compare the new card against 30 to 50 prints obtained from the house, a stack of lifts and photographs about 1.5 inches high. The most recently collected print, from the wall over the body, was on top of the pile. The first one from the pile was the palm print from the wall and it matched. Although excited, the fingerprint examiner followed laboratory procedure that requires verification by another qualified examiner before anyone is notified. After the print was verified, the detectives were contacted during the polygraph and were informed of the confirmed results. It was suggested during a break that the detective should ask the polygrapher to ask Santiago whether he had been in the house. Santiago adamantly denied being in the house and said they would not find his prints there.

Santiago said the print was a mistake and refused to continue with the second polygraph test. He left the room crying and was taken into custody. They wanted a search warrant for Santiago's house and truck, based on the polygraph test, facial hair and palm print. They were looking for a knife, cowboy boots, and clothing he had worn at the party. One might rationalize that the killer, in all likelihood, would get rid of the telltale evidence; but the best policy is not to give up on unlikely clues, obtain a warrant if you can and go looking for those hidden clues. The trace evidence will probably still be there. A search warrant was issued at 1:30 that Friday morning.

The search warrant was served and immediately produced a new pair of blue jeans in the bathroom at Santiago's home (Figure 5.6). The dye had leached from the right knee and there were bloodstains visible. In a closet, size 8½D boots were found with soles that matched the pattern in the footprints at the crime scene. The closet also contained a brown leather jacket with a small amount of suspected blood on a cuff snap (Figure 5.7). Santiago's new red half-ton Chevrolet pickup truck was towed to the laboratory for processing.

Crime scene personnel returned to the laboratory at 5.30 a.m. and put the truck in the locked garage. There were three to four inches of snow in its bed so the garage heaters were turned on to melt the snow and dry the truck for processing. The truck and the area were secured against tampering and the personnel left for breakfast. When they returned, they couldn't believe their eyes. The snow had melted and there was a bent kitchen knife in the truck bed (Figure 5.8). The bloody knife had a brown wooden handle and a blade

Figure 5.6
Blood-stained blue jeans were found in the defendant's house.

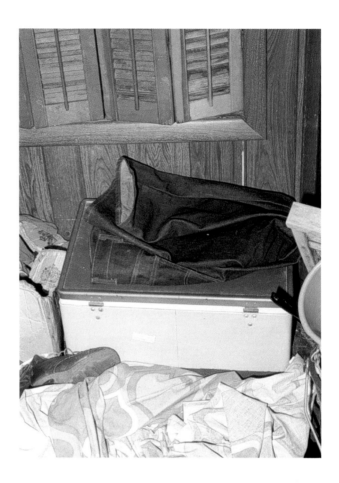

Figure 5.7
Cowboy boots that made the impression on the kitchen floor were found thrown in the defendant's closet. The boot heel supported blood and hair matching the victim.

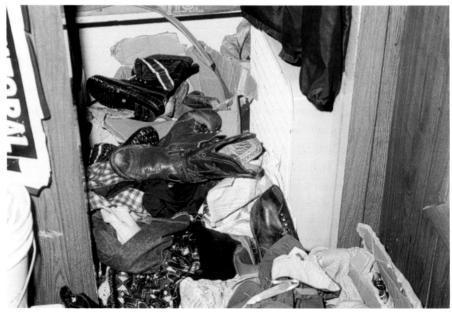

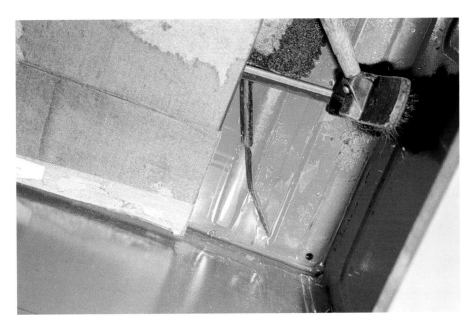

Figure 5.8

When the snow melted from the defendant's truck, the knife from the victim's kitchen was discovered. The knife supported blood and cut pubic hairs that showed it to be the murder weapon.

approximately ⅞ inch wide and 6 inches long, consistent with knife wounds in the victim's chest. Several hair segments were found on the knife and more were recovered from just under the knife on the floor of the truck bed. The next week, the victim's husband identified the knife as the one missing from his kitchen.

LABORATORY ANALYSIS

The amount of blood smeared around the crime scene certainly suggested that one might expect to find blood on the killer's clothing. The pathologist said that, in addition to being slashed, the victim might have been kicked, which was consistent with the greasy, dirty stain on the front of the heel of the right boot. Two pubic hairs were recovered from the stain. The pubic hairs were cut. Chemical and interfacial tube precipitin tests on the stains showed the presence of human blood. Microscopical examination of the two pubic hairs recovered from the bloodstain on the heel and comparison with the victim's pubic hairs showed them to be similar in all respects.

Close inspection of the brown leather jacket from the defendant's residence revealed a red-brown stain surrounding the snap of the right sleeve cuff. Chemical, serological and immunohematological tests indicated the blood to be type A, the same type as the victim and unlike the suspect who was type O. Red brown crusted stains were noted on the right lower leg and left knee area of the new Levi's blue jeans recovered from the Santiago residence. Chemical and serological tests showed the presence of human blood. Absorption elution tests on the human blood from the left leg indicated the blood to be group A, and indicated the presence of M and rh″(E) blood group factors, all consistent with the victim's blood, although approximately 9 per cent of the population have these factors.

Chemical and serological tests, using Lattes crust and absorption elution techniques, on the blade of the knife recovered from the suspect's pickup truck showed the presence of type A human blood. Three pubic hairs recovered from the hilt of the knife and one pubic hair recovered from under the knife in the pickup were shown to be microscopically similar in all respects to the pubic hair of the victim. Just as those found on the victim's nightgown and the boot heel, the pubic hairs were cut.

Michigan courts, at the time, were concerned about the prejudicial effect of blood typing where the frequency of occurrence of the blood groups was relatively large. The admission of the blood evidence was not assured, although the courts subsequently upheld its use in Santiago's trial. Blood identification today provides a great deal more proof than it did twenty years ago, but the collateral trace evidence in this case illustrates how, even without DNA evidence, the case can be proved.

At the time the victim's nightgown (hospital gown) was first inspected at the crime scene, an apparent fabric impression was noted on the chest area, an impression in blue dye in a pattern typical of denim and unlike the plain weave fabric of the nightgown. There must have been contact between the victim's chest area and the perpetrator's blue jeans.

Upon finding Santiago's blue jeans, it was noted that the right knee area alone was faded, unlike the rest of the blue jeans. The blue jeans were tested with water and shown to fade readily and to leave a blue fabric impression when pressed against white cloth. The blue jeans had apparently never been washed. The size and pattern of the impression made by the blue jeans when kneeling onto a test surface were consistent with the blue fabric impression found on the victim's nightgown.

Using a lifting tape, foreign fibers were collected from the new blue jeans. Microscopical examination of the tape revealed several blue-green acrylic fibers similar to the fibers composing the victim's blue-green bathrobe. Each of the matching fibers was excised from the lifting tape, remounted on microscope slides, and compared using a stereomicroscope, polarizing microscope, and comparison microscope. The questioned and known fibers were similar with regards to color, diameter, shape, birefringence, sign of elongation, relative refractive index, cross-sectional shape, and delustering. Today, the acrylic fibers would probably also be compared using fluorescence microscopy, microspectrophotometry, and infrared microspectroscopy.

THE LIFTING TAPE

Essentially unchanged from the 19th century, the techniques for collecting trace evidence include: (1) visual search and picking microtraces directly, (2) beating garments in a bag, (3) filtered vacuum sweepings, (4) shaking, brushing, brooming or scraping of garments over clean paper, (5) lifting with an adhesive substrate like tape, (6) combing, and (7) clipping. From the beginning of the 20th century, forensic scientists were probably already looking to Hans Gross for inspiration regarding methods of collecting trace evidence. Dr. Gross was Professor of Criminology at the University of Prague and seems to have written the first book of police forensic investigations, originally titled *Handbuch für Unter-suchungsrichter als System der Kriminalistik*, published in the last quarter of the 19th century, a book from which all subsequent criminalistics texts seem to emanate. He put garments in a closed paper bag and beat the bag with rods or beaters called tapettes, used by housekeepers to clean draperies and upholstery. The dust particles accumulated in the bottom of the bag. Though primitive, Gross thought it was certainly much preferable to the brushing process, which extracts dust only to scatter it away. Later, Locard (1930) recommended that microtraces that can be seen be collected directly using forceps and needles and placed in a folded paper packet. He recommended collecting diffused unseen dust by vacuuming or by scraping loose material downward on to a glass plate coated with glycerin.

The concept of using an adhesive coated film for fingerprint lifting was known at the beginning of the 20th century. Dubois, a Brazilian, first described lifting of latent fingerprints developed with powder in 1899 using a lifter with a tacky surface that was pressed against the print and pulled away. The adhesive surface was then covered with a thin film of celluloid (the backer) which protected the lifted powder and pattern. Originally, the lifter was made from a mixture of gelatin and glucose, replaced soon thereafter by rubber. As with tape, the fingerprint powder particles adhere to the sticky surface of the rubber lifter and thus transfer the pattern of the fingerprints (Svensson and Wendel 1965).

Even before Locard published his studies on dust, he delved into the identification of forged fingerprints. One way to fake a print is to collect an original latent fingerprint from an innocent surface and claim it was collected from another incriminating surface, i.e. a transferred powdered lift. Locard reported that the transferred powdered lift could often be debunked by study of the microscopic debris in the lift with the fingerprint (Moenssens 1971). A recent example illustrates how Locard was right (Bisbing 1989). A fingerprint was developed on a windowsill and subsequently identified as the defendant's in a home invasion case. It was postulated that the lift may have been collected from the vehicle in which the defendant was arrested and searched, instead of from the windowsill as the police claimed. The windowsill was marble and the

Figure 5.9

Marble dust on a latent fingerprint lift that showed that the finger-print was lifted from the windowsill rather than the car. Photomicrograph is taken with crossed polars showing the interference colors of the particles.

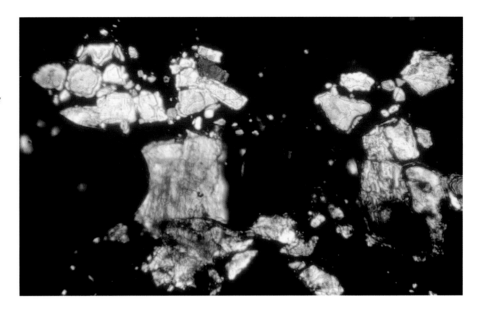

innocent surface was painted. No paint particles were found anywhere on the tape, but in a portion of the tape where black fingerprint powder had apparently accumulated in a crack in the windowsill surface, calcium carbonate crystals were abundant, similar in all respects to marble dust (Figure 5.9). The tape lifted the fingerprint pattern, detected the location of the crack in the windowsill and recovered particles for identification, as expected.

Sedimentologists use lacquer and acetate peels in an analogous way to replicate sedimentary structures and patterns and to collect specimens for microscopical study. The lacquer method was developed by von Dr Ehrhard Voigt, Halle/Saale, Germany, in 1932 to salvage vertebrates from German Eocene lignite deposits, including the hair of vertebrates, red blood corpuscles of a lizard, and soft parts of insects (Voigt 1938). Besides the application in paleontology, Voigt also used small micropeels in forensic investigations to detect blood traces, textile fragments, hair and fingerprints which were collected for microscopical study. Acetate peels are used in a similar way (McCrone 1963). The film adheres to the rock and when peeled off replicates the surface structure while small amounts of soft surface rock material remains stuck to the peel in a manner that accurately records color as well as texture. The peels can be used like photographic negatives to make enlarged photographs of the patterns and the particulate material can be excised for analysis.

Fortunately, an invention spawned in the automobile industry ultimately produced the transparent lifting tape required by the criminalist. Scotch™ brand paint masking tape was developed about 1925 to allow the automobile manufacturers to spray paint in a straight line. The masking tape was well established in 1930 when a new tape was brought to market which was clear. The new

Scotch™ tape was almost invisible and had a backing and adhesive so clear that it could be used to mend pages in books without affecting readability, lift fingerprints, and permit a microscopical examination of particles embedded in the adhesive.

Midway through the 20th century, it was Max Frei-Sulzer, of the Zurich Police Department Crime Laboratory (Frei-Sulzer 1951, 1965) who apparently first recommended collecting trace evidence completely invisible to the naked eye by pressing ordinary Scotch tape to the surface where microtraces were suspected to be present, that is, in "hot zones." After collecting the microtraces, his advice was to fold the used part upon a clean strip, after which you get a document from the scene of the crime in which it is even possible to study the distance between the single particles and the pattern of particles, if they are lifted like a fingerprint impression. He also explained that the tape with the lifted microscopic traces is never opened, so that any loss of evidence and any contamination with foreign dust are avoided. Instead, if an examination under a stereomicroscope shows interesting details or microtraces, a few of them are cut or punched out, while the remainder of the tape is left intact for additional study if warranted.

The folding-over of the lift tape upon itself, as described by Frei-Sulzer, is usually discouraged, although it is easy enough to make it useful, particularly at the crime scene. Admittedly, this procedure makes it a little more difficult to remove trace evidence for subsequent analysis. The particles are more easily recovered when sandwiched between tape and a plastic sheet or glass slide than between two strips of adhesive tape. There simply is less adhesive to deal with. Therefore, where possible, the tape lift should be stuck onto clear (transparent) plastic sheets or glass slides. On the other hand, if the tape has lost all its tack and does not adhere to the backer or slide, backing the lifting tape onto another piece of tape might be prudent in order to prevent subsequent contamination. The additional adhesive from the backing tape encapsulates the particles and prevents their loss and fully covers the adhesive, preventing extraneous particles from falling on exposed adhesive that might result from the tape loosening from the backer.

The lifting tape is a speedy and convenient way to collect trace evidence for the following reasons: (1) removes foreign particles efficiently, (2) removes minimal background material, (3) permits sampling of areas of choice, (4) prevents subsequent contamination, (5) facilitates the initial identification of particles, and (6) permits particles to be easily removed for subsequent analysis. One of the distinct advantages is the resultant transparent sample medium. On no account should the tape be stuck onto paper or cardboard, although for fingerprints it is a common practice. Being able to use a transmitted light base or different colored backgrounds when viewing the tapes with a stereomicroscope sometimes facilitates the detection of the microtraces. Likewise, the transparent backer allows the use of a polarizing or other compound microscope with transmitted light for initial characterization of particles.

It can be seen that for over one hundred years, microtraces have been collected with sticky tape for the same two reasons: (1) reproduction of patterns of particles and (2) recovery of particles for subsequent analysis. The best example is the use of transparent tape to collect dusted fingerprints, which is a collection of small particles in a pattern. Tape is also routinely used around the world to collect textile fibers from clothing, a technique for which it is best known to the trace evidence examiner. Fibers are really just special particles that are collected with tape usually for the sole purpose of subsequent identification and comparison with possible sources. Sometimes the latent print lift is used to collect particles for analysis if there is interest in the nature of the material creating the fingerprint or in the nature of the surface from which the print was lifted. Sometimes the fiber lift is used to reproduce patterns if there is an apparent fabric impression.

The use of transparent lifting tape to collect fingerprints and fiber evidence is a relatively routine procedure in criminal investigations. Nevertheless, there are other examples where opaque lifting tape is also invaluable. The analysis of gunshot residues (GSR) using scanning electron microscopy and x-ray spectrometry (SEM/EDS/WDS) has proven to be a valuable addition to the trace evidence arsenal. The basic principle upon which the technique depends is that small particles characteristically left as a residue after a weapon is fired can be collected using adhesive coated SEM stubs. Today, opaque conductive carbon-filled double-sided tape disks are used on the stubs. The subsequent analysis is performed in the SEM directly on the adhesive surface; and particles unique to GSR are identified by their morphology and chemical composition. For example, if a replicate taping is used to collect particles from the interior of a vehicle thought to have been involved in a drive-by shooting, the number and pattern of particles can be determined and thereby evidence regarding the location of the shooter. In other words, gunshot residue particles are collected by tape either for determining their concentration and pattern or for the analysis of individual particles, the same reason lifting tape is always used.

The technique of lifting fingerprints illustrates the procedure required to collect trace evidence as well, whether lifting a footwear impression, a fabric impression or individual particles. After the impression or debris is discovered, an identification tag for the lift is prepared upon which is written: (1) case number, (2) date, (3) time, (4) name of person collecting lift, (5) object from which print is being lifted, and (6) location of object, including distances from landmarks and orientation directions (up and down or compass direction). The tag can then be shown right side up in any close-up photographs taken of the evidence in situ and incorporated in the subsequent lift as an identification tag.

To lift a print or impression, use 1.5 inch wide transparent tape, wider if for a shoe print or a 1:1 replication lift, or lay strips parallel to each other to cover the area of interest. Strip off a length of tape and attach the loose end to the surface near the impression so that the tape can be positioned over the developed print or fabric impression. Press down firmly, starting at the end attached to the surface and apply even pressure across the length and width of the tape. After the print is completely covered by the tape, lift it off with a smooth, even movement, holding the still attached roll. The powder, fibers and other particles will adhere to the tape. Stick the loose end to a clean surface like a clip board, slide a clear plastic backer under the tape, and again starting at the affixed end apply pressure toward the other end still attached to the roll. Place the identification tag, which might already have been used in a photograph, between the tape and the backer in a position where it does not interfere with the print or microtraces, just before the remaining tape is pressed onto the backer. If need be, the tape can be further pressed onto the backer using a pencil eraser.

As previously described for acetate peels, the transparent lift can be used as a negative for photographic contact prints or enlargements if required, used for pattern comparisons directly, or searched under a stereomicroscope for micro-traces (Bridges 1942; Myre 1974).

Forensic scientists usually devise their own ways to use the tape for collecting trace evidence. Just as one example, a paint roller with masking tape backed around it was first used by the author in about 1972 to collect hair and fiber evidence. A search was conducted for black polyester sweater fibers on the black lining of an overcoat, black acrylic lining fibers on the sweater, short curly black wig fibers on the outer surface of the shaggy black wool overcoat, and curly black hairs on all the items, all in hopes of reconstructing a disguise used by a bank robber. Tape was the only way to detect the foreign fibers so the traditional lint roller used to clean suits and uniforms was considered. Rather than requisi-tioning one, the device was made from an ordinary paint roller frame and ordinary masking tape. Because black hairs and fibers were the target materials, the white background of the masking tape provided sufficient contrast. After the fibers and hairs were collected, the roller was searched under a stereo-microscope and hairs and fibers of interest were collected from the surface of the tape and mounted on slides. Shortly after this, transparent tape was used for lifting. As a consequence, due to differences in pliability between the masking tape and the transparent book tape, the paint roller no longer worked well. Thereafter, the tape back was reversed over the roll from which it was stripped forming a roller of sorts with the sticky side out (Figure 5.10). Three-inch wide book tape was used most often, although the roller can be formed with 1–2 inch wide fingerprint lifting tape just as easily. Scotch 3M No. 845 Book Tape in

Figure 5.10

Transparent tape roll used as a roller device to collect microtraces from the surface of the sweater.

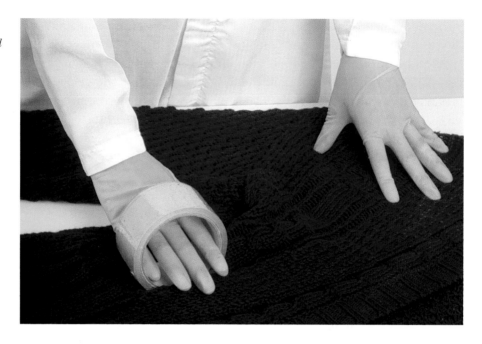

3-inch wide rolls and Scotch Clear Plastic Tape in 1.5-inch wide rolls works very well.

Other means have been described for using the tape or adhesive sheets with roller devices (Grieve and Garger 1981; Fong 1984; Choudhry 1988, 1989; Flinn 1992; Swinton 1999). Some of the devices require quite complicated preparation procedures and at times during either the preparation of the device or the subsequent search and recovery of fibers, the adhesive surface is exposed excessively, thereby risking contamination. The principal advantages of the adhesive rolling method are the avoidance of dust, ease of search, and convenience of storing the rollings. An additional advantage is that, in favorable circumstances, bunches of fibers representing several types of fibers and colors are transferred to the adhesive as clusters and remain as such until excised for analysis, more like a replication lift.

In order to collect the trace evidence, the roller or larger piece of tape is lightly rubbed over the surface, either in a sweeping motion across the surface in the area of interest or patted onto the surface in sequential steps. Particles are recovered from the surface with each pass of the tape. The tape is used in this manner until it loses its tack and particles no longer adhere. After an area has been swept or patted down, the tape is unfastened from the roll, straightened out, and placed sticky side down on a clear plastic sheet or on to another length of clean tape from the same roll. In any event, whether the microtraces are lifted like a fingerprint or collected with a roller, after the tape has been securely affixed to a backer, the particles collected are forever secured and prevented from further loss or contamination. Under no circumstances should the adhesive surface remain exposed or ever be opened and exposed again unless it can be assured that the room, bench, tools, and personnel are particle free, as in a cleanroom.

Sweeping with strips of tape or roller devices in localized areas helps define where the microtraces were found, but they do not reproduce precise locations or patterns. Patterns, like fingerprints, are replicated with a single application of the tape and immediate transfer to a backing. For trace evidence such as foreign fibers on clothing, vehicle interiors and furniture upholstery, it is sometimes valuable to replicate the location and patterns of the microtraces so that there is one-to-one correspondence between the particles recovered with the tape and the exact location from which they originated on the item taped. Michael Grieve of the Bundeskriminalamt Kriminaltechnisches Institut in Wiesbaden, Germany, describes the technique which was apparently first used in Germany in the early 1980s by Dr. D. Neubert-Kirfel of the Landeskriminalamt Nordrhein-Westfalen, Dusseldorf (Robertson and Grieve 1999). The entire surface of interest is covered with strips of tape and each piece is numbered, photographed, and mapped in order to allow the exact location of each tape to be documented (Figure 5.11). When the tapes are pulled from the surface, the 1:1 taping method records the precise original location of all the microtraces.

Ideally, the method should be used right at the crime scene before anything is moved. In cases of homicide, bodies and the area surrounding the body are

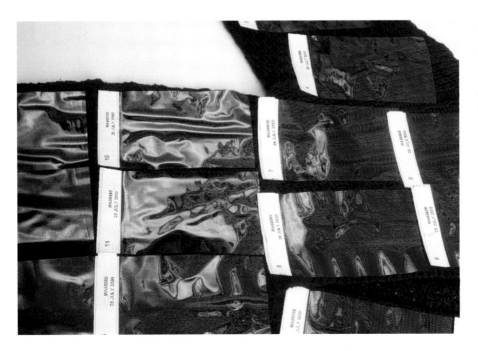

Figure 5.11
A 1:1 taping of the sweater. The surface is covered with separate pieces of lifting tape. Each piece is numbered and the location is recorded. Later each tape is searched separately for trace evidence and the types and numbers of particles compared with those collected from other locations on the sweater.

good candidates for replication taping. The microtrace replication technique is the best way to quantitatively evaluate fiber and microtrace transfer. It is sometimes possible to tell from the number of fibers and the patterns something about the area of most intense contact, about the different garments worn by an assailant, or about from which side the attack occurred. For many cases, the number of tapes obtained is greater than a roller device, which then seems to increase the amount of work required to search them for evidence; however, the actual number of microtraces that require analysis may not be greater than taping with a single tape over the same surface.

Although trace evidence is usually used in criminal investigation, another interesting application of the microtrace replication technique is the investigation of the Turin Shroud. It may be the most contentious taping yet; even more contentious than the Guy Paul Morin tapes. In 1973, while Max Frei-Sulzer was authenticating photographs of the Turin Shroud taken in 1969, he noticed that the surface of the Shroud was covered with minute dust particles. He therefore asked for permission to remove some of the particles for analysis. On the night of 23 November, with the Shroud still hanging vertically in the frame used for the television exposition, Frei took his samples from the bottom zone to the left and right, and from the side strip. His method was absurdly simple: he pressed small pieces of clean adhesive tape onto the surface of the linen, then sealed these into plastic envelopes and put them into the modest satchel that he carried constantly with him (Wilson 1978).

John H. Heller (1983), who writes as though he was actually there, describes how Max Frei-Sulzer again was asked to collect sticky tape samples from the Shroud during the STURP investigation in 1978. Frei-Sulzer took out a Scotch tape container like the kind one buys in Woolworth's. He had on a pair of cotton gloves that the team had brought. He pulled off a piece of tape with the gloved fingers and without any reference chart began putting on pieces of tape and ripping them off. After some confusion and contention, Frei-Sulzer gave up and stomped out of the room, glowering.

In contrast to what Max Frei-Sulzer had done, an individually designed adhesive-tape applicator was constructed by Ray Rogers for removal of tiny samples of the Shroud's body and blood images. He designed a device to exert uniform pressure on the tapes, a box to store the tapes as they were taken and arranged to obtain a quantity of special tape which used a special pure hydrocarbon adhesive formulated by the 3M Company on special polyester tape. There had been considerable discussion as to what kind of adhesive to put on the tape. As soon as each tape lift was removed from the Shroud, the tape was affixed sticky-side downward on to a glass microscope slide. Careful notes were made of the points from which they had been removed and then the slides were packed into containers to await transport. The procedure was designed to be completely non-destructive to the linen. Wherever a sample was taken, physical measurements were made and the locations recorded on a grid (Wilson 1988).

Not only has Walter C. McCrone disagreed with just about everyone else's conclusions regarding what the tapes showed, he also disliked the tape. Dr McCrone (1996) wrote how fortunate it was that Ray Rogers of Los Alamos was strongly in favor of the Shroud tape sampling. However, according to McCrone, the polyester tape chosen by Rogers was inferior optically to almost any other possible tape. He thought the samples taken by Max Frei-Sulzer were far superior from an optical point of view.

Regardless of the contention, the lift tape proved invaluable as one means to study the Turin Shroud. Particles were recovered for identification in a quantitative way from different areas of the item, and the tape lifts provided a permanent document of the dust particles, pollen grains and paint pigments, which could be studied over and over again for years without fear of subsequent contamination or loss.

Once microtraces have been collected and sealed within the tape adhesive on a backer, the tape will normally need to be searched for fibers or particles of interest, the microtraces characterized in some way, and some of them recovered from the adhesive for further study. There are a variety of ways to search the tape and study the particles; there are ways in which the tape itself can be used to facilitate the microscopical examination; and there are different ways to excise the particles for subsequent analysis.

None of the commercially available tapes are perfectly suited for use as a particle mountant for polarized light microcopy (PLM) due to anisotropy of the backing and the not so useful refractive index of the adhesive. Nevertheless, many examinations can be made directly through the tape before demounting hairs, fibers, and particles for further study. For example, Crocker (1998) describes the value of transparent tape as a mountant to study the cuticular scale features of certain animal hairs. When hairs are covered with tape and viewed with bright-field transmitted light, the scale pattern and other surface details are well resolved and clearly visible.

In a similar vein, Iwamoto and Gaudette (2000) describe a method of preparing hair samples for morphological examination, which makes use of a polyester lifting sheet developed by Lintec Co. of Japan. The transparent sheet is constructed of a 100 μm thick polyester sheet adhering to a 40 μm thick polypropylene cover sheet. Hair samples are placed on the adhesive surface of the polyester sheet and then covered by the polypropylene cover sheet. Specimens prepared in this manner can be studied microscopically using either transmitted or reflected light. The scales and other features are easily viewed. The hairs can be easily removed from the sheet for subsequent DNA analysis if required. The wide sheets were originally designed for collecting footprints at crime scenes and come in 10 m × 1 m rolls.

In those instances where smaller particles need to be scrutinized, the tapes can be searched with the aid of a stereomicroscope. A transmitted light base is useful on occasion and different colored backgrounds can be used depending on the color of the microtraces of interest. Sometimes a grid is placed under the tapes to facilitate the searching process and to record the location of interesting particles. Interesting particles can be marked and numbered with a permanent felt marker on the backer side. In order to recover the particles, the tapes are turned over and the excisions are made through the tape side, thereby not messing the marks.

If a large number of tapes with thousands of particles and fibers need to be searched for materials of interest, painstaking manual and visual searching using a stereomicroscope can be time-consuming, tedious and ultimately fatiguing. Fortunately, there are instruments available for automated unattended searching of the tapes, which take advantage of image analysis software and motorized microscope stages. For example, Foster+Freeman's FibreFinder® is a color scanner that uses several wavelengths of light and records the position of each fiber of a selected color. While operating for only a few minutes, an actual size schematic print out of each tape showing the position and shape of the chosen color fiber is produced which is used by the microscopist to relocate the fibers of interest. The color scanner only measures colors and shapes. The machine cannot distinguish synthetic from natural fibers, define their cross-sectional shape or whether they are delustered or not. Experienced microscopists can rapidly sort the fibers using these additional characteristics. Therefore, the image analysis system is only useful in those rare cases where too many tapes need to be scanned in too short a period of time. Normally, manual and visual scanning is more efficient in the long run.

On a smaller scale, if short strips of tape are used to pick up small samples of particles, the adhesive side can be pressed against a glass cover slip. In other words, a thin glass cover slip is used as a backer. The cover slip is placed on a microscope slide sandwiching the tape between the cover slip and the slide. Solvent is allowed to pass under the cover slip thereby clearing the tape and adhesive to facilitate the microscopical study of the particles collected. The particles are now in a softened adhesive nearest the cover slip, between the cover slip and the tape film. In this way, the tape is not nearly as bothersome when the particles are studied with a microscope.

Finally, in many instances, the particles of interest need to be excised from the tape lift and analyzed. John Gustav Delly (1969), retired from McCrone Research Institute, recommended a long time ago that particles requiring identification that are received embedded in the adhesive of transparent tape can be mounted for microscopical study by placing one or two drops of benzene on the adhesive and using the side of a microspatula or needle to scoop up the sample. The sample can then be placed directly on a slide and covered with a cover glass. Since the refractive index of most adhesives is 1.49–1.50 and that of benzene is 1.50, the index of the resulting medium will be somewhere between 1.49 and 1.50. Alternatively, the adhesive can be rinsed off and the particles mounted in a different medium of choice. Some tapes are partly soluble in a variety of common solvents, which makes recovery of small particles easier.

Another method for recovering fibers and other particulates from the tape utilizes a "flap."[2] The top layer of tape is sliced along the imaginary lines of the equal sides of an isosceles triangle, where the apex of the triangle is positioned over the particle of interest, leaving the base attached. A small drop of solvent is placed at the apex of the triangle and allowed to diffuse into the adhesive, thereby releasing the triangular flap from the backing and the fiber or particle of interest. The adhesive and fiber are scooped from under the flap and transferred to a clean microscope slide. The triangular flap is replaced and secured with a piece of transparent tape to prevent subsequent contamination. Alternatively, a punch can be used to excise the particles of interest. The punch produces a manageable sized disk, which includes the tape, adhesive, particle of interest, and backing. After punching out the sample, the disk is manipulated with solvents and probes in order to recover the particles of interest. When the particle is recovered from the tape adhesive, the remaining adhesive can be rinsed off with a suitable solvent and the fiber or particle mounted semi-permanently on the microscope slide for subsequent microscopical study or analysis. The microtrace is now ready for identification and comparison. Other microtraces remain secure in the tape lift available and ready for future study.

[2] The author is indebted to John Funk at the Centre of Forensic Sciences in Toronto for this techniques.

CONTAMINATION PREVENTION AND CONTROL

Throughout an investigation and trial, considerable weight will be placed on the results of the examination of the trace evidence. Therefore, it is essential, obviously, that the samples represent the actual samples present at the time of the crime and there must be no possibility of one sample becoming contaminated with any other. The best collection techniques are useless if they cannot be relied upon to protect the evidence from contamination. The lift tape is very efficient; it will pick up the tiniest particle but the accidental transfer of small particles between the work environment and the tape is very likely. At the same time, the lift tape can protect the microtraces from subsequent contamination. In general, prevention of contamination is based on awareness of potential microtraces, minimizing the chances for accidental transfer, and the use of controls.

One needs only to review the case of Guy Paul Morin in Toronto, Canada to better understand the consequences from contamination of lifting tapes (Kaufman 1998). Lifting tapes used to collect foreign fibers from clothing that associated Morin with the victim in that case were shown to have been contaminated with the questioned fibers while in the laboratory at the Centre of Forensic Sciences. The association between the defendant and victim was based on somewhat unusual similar questioned fibers found on both the victim and defendant's clothing. The original source of either the associated questioned fibers or the source of the contaminating fibers was never discovered, although an investigation seemed to suggest that the contaminate was from a garment worn by one of the laboratory technicians. At the time, the laboratory had neither a consistent practice regarding contamination prevention nor any control tapes to assist in reconstructing the events. Furthermore, although the inquiry report is unclear, it appears that the adhesive of the lifting tapes was periodically exposed to the laboratory environment and the technicians, thereby permitting the contamination. If the tapes are placed sticky side up and loosely covered with an acetate sheet that is periodically removed to recover more fibers, it is no wonder that the tapes may be regularly contaminated.

Contamination prevention begins at the crime scene. All crime scenes are protected in the same general way. The scene must be left as a frozen section in space, time, form, and context. The action needs to be stopped so that nothing foreign is introduced, nothing is destroyed, and nothing inadvertently removed. Contamination is prevented by taking measures against the five major contaminators: weather, relatives, friends and associates, the curious, and officials. Only the weather cannot think. If everyone else on the list would think of footprints first and trace evidence second, more crime scenes would be better protected. When the scene is adequately protected, the trace evidence will be observed or discovered in place, photographed, measured and mapped, and expertly collected with a short chain of custody and with very much less chance of contamination.

Personnel who participate in the processing and collection of evidence should wear clothing that protects themselves from contamination at the scene and protects the scene from contamination by the investigator. Uniforms, coveralls, or laboratory coats should be worn at all times by personnel at the scene until the trace evidence has been discovered and recovered. The clothing should be clean, free from excessive microtraces and of known composition. Hands can be protected by rubber gloves.

People at the scene (victims, witnesses, and suspects) need to be physically separated and interviewed separately. This is a classic investigative technique to ensure independent stories, but it is also valuable to prevent cross-contamination after the incident has occurred. Ideally, the police should use different interviewers, conduct interviews of victims and suspects in different rooms, or, at least, using different chairs.

One of the extra values of the lift tape is its role in contamination control and detection. Michael Grieve (1983) introduced the concept of using the tape as a control procedure. Control tapes can be collected from areas where contact is not expected to determine if the foreign fibers or other microtraces are ubiquitous or concentrated in the "hot zones," as Frei-Sulzer would have described them. For example, control tapes can be taken from the investigator's clothing and witnesses who were not in contact with the principals. Control tapings from chairs, desks, police cars, emergency room tables, would be useful, although admittedly time-consuming. Elimination of potential contamination from the legitimate environment of the people involved will greatly enhance the value of any subsequent trace evidence associations. When the microscopist cannot say with certainty that a particular suite of fibers or a type of soil could not have originated from the defendant's own legitimate environment, the opinion that it could have originated from the victim's clothing or the crime scene loses much of its value. Worse would be a claim of contamination by the police investigators, when no preventive measures or controls were taken to counteract the claim.

The laboratory provides a much better environment for collection of trace evidence, but it should be emphasized that contamination at the search stage is still a very great risk. Once in the laboratory, contamination is usually caused either by airborne particles, by secondary transfer during laboratory processing or by primary transfer from the person or clothing of laboratory personnel.

Distance and barriers can prevent airborne transfer. For example, items of clothing from victim and suspect should be searched in separate rooms (separated by walls and doors) or at least on separate tables (separated by some distance). Secondary transfer involves the exchange of particles from a contaminated surface during contact rather than the exchange of particles from the original materials themselves, which is referred to as a primary transfer. Secondary transfer seems most likely to occur when the surface is dirty, that is, when foreign particles are present in abundance and loosely bound. Therefore, eliminating contact between a dirty surface and the evidence can prevent secondary transfers. The dirty surface could be the laboratory bench or the laboratory coat of the person processing the evidence. Either the contact is simply prohibited or, if contact is allowed, the surface is cleaned first. Primary transfer from the processors is prevented by using gloves, laboratory gowns, and constant vigilance. Control lift tapes should be collected simultaneously with the processing and contiguous with the items processed, that is, at the same time and place as the items being processed.

Based on these general concepts, some simple suggestions might help prevent contamination in the laboratory (Pounds 1975). When handling evidence, the examiner must be clothed in a garment that is clean and of known composition. Generally, the questioned exhibits should be searched before any controls are unpacked. Never allow suspect and victim garments to rest on the same surface. Presumably, the individual items will have arrived in the laboratory packaged in separate paper bags; and thereafter, the victim's and suspect's items should be processed in separate, specially designed processing rooms, like cleanrooms with controlled air pressure, humidity, and temperature, and where the air is circulated through HEPA filters. Different tables should be used for different garments. Examining tables must be clean. New underlying paper should be used for each garment. Specimens collected should be immediately covered. Tape lifts should be immediately sealed onto a backer before another garment is processed. Control tapes should be used in the laboratory to assure that microtraces thought to be from a specific item are not contaminants from the laboratory environment or a previous sample.

In the laboratory, forensic scientists can design the controls necessary to assure everyone that contamination could not occur while the evidence is in the laboratory's custody. Controls might include something as simple as lift tapes from the table or examiner's clothing. Alternatively, a piece of felt or other passive substrate can be placed on the table near where the evidential items are being processed. Before each item is processed, a tape lift is collected from the passive substrate. Before an association is made between microtraces collected from the evidential item with microtraces from another source, all of the control tapes must be free of the source material. If they are not, you have to wonder where they came from and why they are there.

After processing of the items from one source, the tools, table, room, etc. should be thoroughly cleaned and gowns changed. Control tapes are then collected to demonstrate the cleanliness of the processing environment. In other words, the processing rooms are controlled in the same way as instruments are controlled. With instruments, records are kept of maintenance, repair, calibrations, standards tested, and the results from blanks. With rooms, the control tapes should be evaluated for microtraces of interest, the results recorded in a log, and the samples kept for future reference as part of the laboratory's quality assurance program. If questions are asked later regarding whether a particular sample could have been contaminated by a previous case processed in the same room or by the same people, the control tapes taken following the previous sample and/or just prior to the sample in question can be searched for the microtraces of interest. If none are found then the answer is no. If the control tapes are loaded with particles just like those associated in the subsequent case, there is a problem. The consequence of contamination is too great to be ignored. Measures must be in place to prevent and control the possibility of accidental transfer of microtraces in the laboratory.

CONCLUSION

Frederico Santiago was tried for murder the following winter. For some inexplicable reason, the trial and deliberations dragged on into the early spring, longer than a typical murder trial in the Midwest. Expert testimony provided a plethora of evidence associating the defendant with the crime, including the following.

The palm print on the kitchen wall over the victim was identified as the defendant's and gained pre-eminent importance when the polygraph examiner elicited the statement from the defendant that he had never been to the victim's residence, did not know where she lived, did not know the victim, and "even my brother knows I have never been there". Court displays were prepared illustrating the palm print and footwear identifications. Although the palm print was distorted and initially thought to be not displayable, extra efforts were taken with the photographs until each matching minutia could be numbered. The defense's expert reportedly could not identify the palm print during his initial re-analysis of the lifts, but when he was shown the display by the defense attorney prior to being called to the witness stand, he could see the identification. To the consternation of the defense attorney, the expert said that he would have to identify the print if asked and therefore was going home.

The pattern and accidental marks on the sole of the defendant's cowboy boot matched the pattern and accidental marks in the prints found on the kitchen floor next to the victim's leg, which permitted the expert to testify with certainty that the impression was made by Santiago's boot. In one way, it was more significant than the palm print because, unlike the palm print, there was evidence presented regarding how long the boot print could have been there. The victim's husband testified that the kitchen floor had been washed the day before the murder. Experts did not testify how long the prints were there, but explained that washing with soap and water and scrubbing around would have obliterated them if they had been there before the day of the murder. Upon cross-examination, the defense witness who had examined the footwear impression admitted, when shown the display, that he agreed with all but one individual point and would have to conclude that the impression was made by the defendant's boot. The defense attorney admitted during his closing arguments that the identifications were correct and tried to suggest to the jury that the defendant had forgotten he had been at the crime scene once, a long time ago. He had no explanation for the knife and fabric impression. The images of the knife in the truck and of the blue fabric impression on the front of the victim's nightgown were very persuasive to the jury.

Bloodstains on the blue jeans found in the defendant's residence were grouped in three antigen systems reducing the population frequency to less than 10 per cent. Nearly a year after first being discovered, one of the blood-stains was typed by the defense's expert confirming that the blood could not have originated from the defendant but could be the victim's blood and further reducing the frequency of the types to less than 3 per cent of the population. Today, DNA analysis would likely provide proof that the blood was the victim's.

The defendant was found guilty of first degree murder after 10 weeks of trial and is serving his life sentence in the care of the Michigan Department of Corrections.

REFERENCES

Bisbing, R.E. (1982). In *Forensic Science Handbook*, ed. R. Saferstein, Englewood Cliffs, NJ: Prentice Hall, pp. 184–221.

Bisbing, R.E. (1989) *American Laboratory*, 21(11), 19–24.

Bisbing, R.E. (2000) In *Encyclopedia of Forensic Science*, ed. J.A. Siegel, London: Academic Press.

Bridges, B.C. (1942) *Practical Fingerprinting.* New York: Funk & Wagnalls Company.

Choudhry, M.Y. (1988) *Journal of Forensic Sciences*, 33, 249–253.

Choudhry, M.Y. (1989) US Patent No. 4,805,468, 21 February.

Crocker, E.J. (1998) *The Microscope*, 146, 169–173.

Delly, J.G. (1969) *The Particle Analyst*, Ann Arbor, MI: Ann Arbor Science Publishers.

Faulker, W. (1991) *Intruder in the Dust.* New York: Vantage Books.

Flinn, L.L. (1992) *Journal of Forensic Sciences,* 37, 106–12.

Fong, W. (1984) *Journal of Forensic Sciences*, 29, 55–63.

Frei-Sulzer, M. (1951) *Kriminalistik*, 5, 190–194.

Frei-Sulzer, M. (1965) in *Methods of Forensic Science*, Vol. 4, ed. A.S. Curry, New York: Inter-science Publishers, pp. 143–144.

Grieve, M.C. (1983) *Journal of Forensic Sciences*, 28, 877–887.

Grieve, M.C. and Garger, E.F. (1981) *Journal of Forensic Sciences*, 26, 560–563.

Heller, J.H. (1983) *Report on the Shroud of Turin*, Boston: Houghton Mifflin Co.

Iwamoto, R. and Gaudette, B.D. (2000) *The Microscope*, 48, 45–49.

Kaufman, F. (1998) *The Commission on Proceedings Involving Guy Paul Morin*, Toronto: Ontario Ministry of the Attorney General.

Locard, E. (1930) *The American Journal of Police Science* 1, 276.

McCrone, A.W. (1963) *J. Sediment. Petrol.*, 33, 228–230.

McCrone, W.C. (1996) *Judgement Day for the Turin Shroud,* Chicago: Microscope Publications.

Moenssens, A.A. (1971) *Fingerprint Techniques*, Radnor, PA: Chilton Book Company.

Myre, D.C. (1974) *Death Investigation,* Alexandria, VA: International Association of Chiefs of Police.

Pounds, C.A. (1975) *J. Forensic Science Society* 15, 127–132.

Robertson, J. and Grieve, M. (1999) *Forensic Examination of Fibres*, 2nd edition, London, Sydney: Taylor & Francis.

Svensson, A. and Wendel, O. (1965) *Techniques of Crime Scene Investigation*, 2nd edition, New York: American Elsevier Publishing Co.

Swinton, S.F. (1999) *Journal of Forensic Sciences*, 44, 1089–1090.

Tessler, A. (1982) *The Saginaw News,* Sunday, 7 February, p. B1–2

Voigt, E. (1938) *Kriminalistik, Monatschfte für die gesamte kriminalistische Wissenschaft u. Praxis*, 12, 265–269.

Wilson, I. (1978) *The Shroud of Turin, The Burial Cloth of Jesus Christ?,* Garden City, NY: Doubleday & Company.

Wilson, I. (1988) *The Mysterious Shroud,* Garden City, NY: Doubleday & Company.

CHAPTER 6

"ONLY CIRCUMSTANTIAL EVIDENCE"

Scott Ryland and Max M. Houck

INTRODUCTION

April 1995 in Central Florida brought with it the death of Jenny Kilborn.[1] Jenny, a vibrant nine-year-old, was abducted from her apartment complex parking lot, strangled and her lifeless body clad only in her T-shirt, shorts, underwear and a thirty-gallon black plastic garbage bag was dumped near a local residential water pumping station. The lack of eyewitnesses to the abduction resulted in a suspect list that included apartment complex acquaintances as well as family members. Jenny's mother, who was inside the apartment, last saw her daughter playing in the parking area in front of the building. When she discovered her absence, she reported it to the police. As interviews and the search began, an anonymous 911 call to the local police dispatcher reported the location of Jenny's body. Of course, the conversation was recorded. This call further focused investigators' attention on people who knew Jenny.

From the forensic viewpoint, the case was a challenge. As will be seen as the story unfolds, there was an absence of the classical individualizing types of evidence. No latent fingerprints, no footwear impressions, no blood or other body fluid transfers (e.g. DNA), no bullet and suspected weapon to compare. This daunting challenge for investigators occurs more often than one might expect. In the absence of direct witnesses and individualizing types of physical evidence, they come to rely even more on yet another mute witness, trace evidence. The possibility of trace evidence transfers is always there, as taught by Edmond Locard (1928, 1930). But it is not the favorite of investigators. Conclusions concerning its significance are often not individualizing; that is, there is usually more than one potential source of the material transferred. Multiple types of transfers strengthen evidential significance; however, this makes for labor-intensive and consequently time-consuming examinations resulting in a long wait for results. But in the absence of all other types of individualizing evidence, it is occasionally the only thing left to solve the case. It immediately brings to mind the subtle and astonishing clues discovered and recounted by Sherlock Holmes. However, even trace transfers were potentially tarnished in this instance. All suspects were either related to or known acquaintances of the

[1] All names have been changed.

victim, with potential explanations for trace evidence transfers resulting from routine contact or secondary transfers (e.g. material deposited on one source, then carried by that source to another location and deposited there). Does this negate its value? What is left? What else can be done? These are the thoughts of which investigators' nightmares are made.

THE CRIME SCENE

Jenny was found outside, fully clothed with the garbage bag covering the upper half of her body. The scene was examined for entry or exit evidence. Tire impressions were found in the soil near the area and plaster casts were made. There were no other unusual items discovered in the near vicinity. The body was transported to the morgue where adhering fibers/debris were removed from her skin. The clothing was collected and bagged for submission to the crime laboratory. There was no apparent evidence of sexual intercourse. No foreign body fluids were discovered on her body. The clothing appeared to have an abundance of apparent animal hair clinging to it. The clothing, fibers/debris from Jenny's arms and legs, and the plastic garbage bag were submitted to the laboratory for subsequent examination. Unfortunately, as is usual in this type of case, the family members are immediately suspected. They were interviewed and a roll of black plastic garbage bags was acquired from the truck belonging to the victim's father. A request was made for comparison of the bag on the victim's body with these bags, along with a request to examine the bag from Jenny's body for latent fingerprints. It was further requested that the apparent animal hairs be examined to ascertain the type of animal from which they originated. The recording of the 911 call was studied again and again to determine a profile for the caller and any background noise heard during the male caller's conversation, which might give an indication from where the call was made. Interviews continued.

INVESTIGATION PROGRESS

Laboratory comparison of the bag from Jenny's body with the roll of bags recovered from her father's truck revealed that they were completely different in construction characteristics. Accordingly, it was concluded that they did not have a common origin, that is, the bag over the top of Jenny's body did not come from the roll of black plastic garbage bags in her father's possession. Investigative interrogations also supported the innocence of the parents. Questioning of apartment complex residents disclosed that Jenny had been seen talking with a neighbor in the parking lot prior to her disappearance. The gentleman often used his dog Pepper to gain the attention of the children.

Further interviews focused the investigation on this neighbor, John Cameron. A search warrant for his residence and vehicle was obtained and executed five days following the discovery of Jenny's body. Among the numerous items collected from his apartment were two loose black plastic garbage bags and a partially used box of fifty Glad Quick-Tie (Registered Trademark of First Brands Corporation, Danbury, CT) thirty-gallon garbage bags. Sixteen bags remained in the box. The topmost bag was crumpled, as if it had been removed from the box and then replaced. The tires on his 1994 Chevrolet S-10 Blazer had been replaced three days after Jenny's death. In an attempt to recover them for comparison with the tire impressions recovered from the scene, detectives visited the tire sales store. They learned that after replacement, Cameron had taken all but one of the four replaced tires with him. This tire was turned over to the police by the vendor. Contents of the Blazer were also collected as evidence, including the front and rear floor mats, two blankets, a towel, a spare tire cover, known fiber samples from the floorboard, known fiber samples from the rear seat, and known fiber samples from the rear cargo area. In addition, vacuum sweepings were collected from various areas inside the vehicle. A cloth was taken from Pepper's kennel to represent hair standards for use in comparison with the animal hairs seen on the victim's clothing.

ANALYSIS

Initial laboratory comparison of the bag from the body of the victim with the bags recovered from the suspect's apartment quickly revealed that all but one were of the same brand and type based upon their physical and construction characteristics. Small samples of the bag removed from the victim's body (questioned bag) were taken for subsequent chemical compositional comparisons and it was then processed for latent fingerprints. None of comparative value were discovered. Laboratory examination of the other physical evidence in the case failed to reveal any comparable DNA originating from body fluid transfers. The medical examiner determined Jenny was strangled with no evidence of a sexual assault. The tire impression casts made from tracks at the scene were compared with the one original tire recovered from the suspect's vehicle, but no correspondence was found.

The physical evidence ultimately boiled down to several types. Dog hairs microscopically like those of the suspect's shar-pei dog were found on the victim's clothing. Animal hairs are useful, if frustrating, as trace evidence. Animals shed, some profusely, and this provides a wealth of possible transfer evidence. However, the strongest conclusion a microscopist trained in animal hair comparisons can come to is that the questioned hairs exhibit the same microscopic characteristics as the known animal hairs and that these hairs could have originated from that animal or another animal of the same breed. If the animal is a domesticated pure breed, more potential sources exist than if the animal's heredity is mixed, and this becomes problematic for common breeds of pets. Research is continuing on the application of DNA sequencing to the mitochondrial DNA found in cat and dog hairs and this has the potential to greatly increase the evidentiary value of dog and cat hair in criminal cases.

One peripheral Caucasian pubic hair (originating from just outside the pubic region) was found on the victim's thigh. This hair while unsuitable for microscopic comparison, proved to be valuable in several ways. First, it was de facto evidence of an adult source: a prepubescent child could not have produced that type of hair. Pubic hairs and related body hairs are a product of puberty and their onset is a secondary sexual characteristic. Second, it indicated that involvement of a person who probably self-identified their race as Caucasian, or white. Last, its context with the victim's body was suggestive that the transfer occurred at or about the time of death. Trace materials are lost at a rapid rate with normal activity (Pounds and Smalldon 1975; Robertson *et al.* 1982; Kidd and Robertson 1982). Two attempts were made by independent laboratories to amplify nuclear DNA from the root of the single peripheral pubic hair utilizing STR (short tandem repeat) technology, but to no avail. Finally, mitochondrial DNA was extracted from the hair shaft and compared to that of the suspect by a third independent laboratory mutually agreed upon by the prosecution and the defense. It was found to coincide, but only with a database frequency of approximately 1 in 500.

Several carpet fibers found on the victim's left arm exhibited the same microscopic and optical properties as carpet fibers in the vacuum cleaner bag previously collected from the suspect's apartment. The apartment complex management had professionally cleaned the suspect's apartment and the carpeting had been replaced prior to acquisition of known carpet fiber samples. No records were kept about what kind of carpet had been purchased or what had happened to the old carpet; presumably it sits today in a landfill somewhere. Because no known sample was ever acquired, a confirmatory comparison was never completed. The huge number of these carpet fibers in the vacuum cleaner bag, however, all but assured that these fibers came from the suspect's carpeting. Additionally, carpet-type fibers found in the debris from the victim's right hand and clothing exhibited the same microscopic and optical properties as fibers in the debris from the floor mat of the suspect's vehicle. All of the physical evidence pointed to the suspect having contact with the victim shortly before or at the time of her death.

Finally, a voice print comparison of the recorded 911 telephone call with that of the suspect also yielded positive results.

The prosecuting attorney was concerned over a solely circumstantial evidence case. He was further troubled about the impact of the hair and fiber trace associative evidence, considering it could be argued that the victim did have opportunity to be in contact (either directly or secondarily) with the suspect, his dog, and possibly even his vehicle, in their commonly shared parking lot. This is one of the limitations of trace associative evidence. If the individuals involved in the alleged transfer are known to have been in contact with one another shortly before the incident in question, any transfer discovered may have less significance unless addressing a reconstruction of events. However, if it could be argued that the number of hairs and fibers transferred are inconsistent with secondary transfers, then the potential direct transfers would be the only ones of concern. Could Pepper have innocently had direct contact with Jenny outside the apartment? How did Jenny get carpet fibers like those in the suspect's apartment vacuum cleaner bag on her left arm, considering that adherent fibers on skin are shed relatively quickly? How did Jenny get fibers like those found on the floor mat of the suspect's vehicle on her hand and clothing? Were they perhaps fibers whose source was common to both Cameron's and Jenny's environment? They presented complex questions that would have to be argued in court. On the other hand, if the questioned bag covering Jenny's body came from the box of bags in the suspect's apartment, a direct link to the crime scene would be established. If this link was established, the other trace evidence became far more incriminating. Investigators and the prosecuting attorney requested priority be placed on this comparison.

Detailed comparison of the questioned bag with the loose bags and box of bags in the suspect's possession proceeded by routine procedures reported in the literature by Von Bremen and Blunt (1983), and Castle *et al.* (1994). Comparisons of construction characteristics including colors, dimensions, seam locations, seam styles, tie flap offsets, cut styles, machine extrusion directions, number and relative thickness of laminates, and fold styles were made. The questioned bag was found to be the same type as one of the two loose bags in the apartment as well as the bags remaining in the partially used box of fifty. Further comparison of extrusion die striae between the questioned bag, the loose bag in the suspect's apartment, and the sixteen bags remaining in the box in the suspect's apartment (known bags) revealed that the questioned bag was produced by the same manufacturer, in the same plant, on the same extrusion line, and in approximately the same time frame as the known bags. The underlying principle of this deduction is akin to that of identifying from which gun a bullet was fired. The metal extrusion die from which the plastic film is drawn is much like the barrel of the gun, with its numerous random imperfections changing over a period of time. The striae produced in the extruded plastic film are the result of imperfections in the die, but not in the metal die lips themselves. As Stanko and Attenberger (1996) pointed out, they are the result of deposits of solidified plastic and/or pigment temporarily lodged between the die lips. These deposits come and go as the molten plastic flows through the die, constantly changing in individual dimensions as well as spatial arrangement. The resultant bands imparted to the plastic garbage bag film are referred to as die striae, or die lines.

Although the predominant die striae patterns corresponded between the questioned bag and the known bags, the position of the predominant die striae relative to the top of the bags differed. This indicated the questioned bag was not produced consecutive to the known bags. Furthermore, the bias (slant) of the predominant die striae indicated the bags were produced on a rotating extruder die. This equipment imparts spiraling die striae on the extruded tube of plastic film during the manufacturing process, appearing somewhat like the stripes on a barber pole (Figure 6.1). Sequentially produced bags manufactured by this method have die striae that systematically proceed across the width of the bag. As one studies the striae from one bag to the next, the striae's location changes in a somewhat orderly and predictable fashion. With the knowledge of the position of the striae on the bags and the average change in position of the striae per bag (calculated from the change observed in the known bags), one can reconstruct the sequence of bag manufacture. Subsequent sequencing of the loose bag with those that remained in the box continued as described in Von Bremen and Blunt (1983). Figures 6.2 and 6.3 demonstrate the procedure used to deduce that two bags were missing in the sequence between the loose bag found in the suspect's apartment and those

Figure 6.1
Film extrusion.

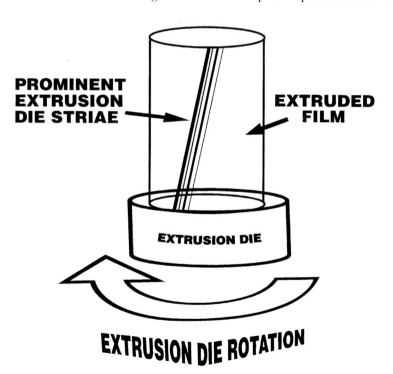

PROMINENT
EXTRUSION
DIE STRIAE

EXTRUDED
FILM

EXTRUSION DIE

EXTRUSION DIE ROTATION

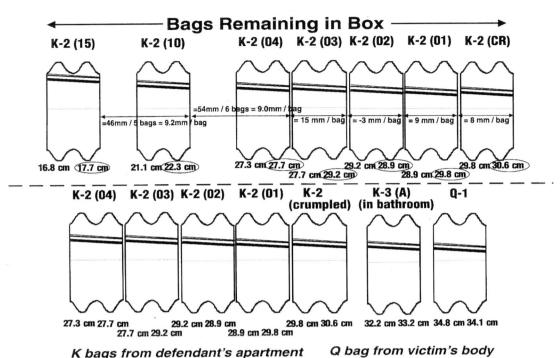

Figure 6.2
Sequencing of bags.

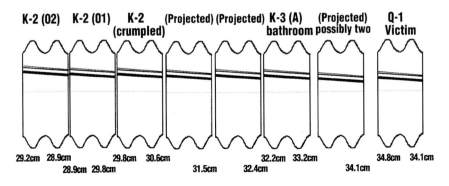

**USING AVERAGE PROJECTED PROCESSION PER BAG OF 0.9 cm
AS CALCULATED FROM K-2 BAGS IN DEFENDANT'S APARTMENT**

Figure 6.3
Sequencing of bags.

remaining in the box. The sixteen bags in the box (designated K-2 in Figures 6.2 and 6.3) were all produced sequentially, each having a direct correspondence of characteristics at the interface of one bag to the next. A further comparison of the position of the predominant die striae relative to the top of the bags between the questioned bag and the loose bag in the apartment indicated the questioned bag was removed in production only one to two bags from the loose bag in the apartment, if it did indeed originate from that box of bags. This is also demonstrated diagrammatically in Figure 6.3.

Since there was not a direct correspondence between the questioned bag and any of the recovered known bags, the obvious question begged to be asked. How many other boxes of Glad Quick-Tie thirty-gallon garbage bags of this style are there which could have been potential sources for the bag found covering Jenny's body? While knowing that answering this question would be difficult, if not impossible, it was decided that an attempt had to be made to assess the number of boxes of bags that may have contained a bag with characteristics like the questioned bag. The prominence of the garbage bag evidence, especially in light of the other evidence available in the case, would compel the question to be asked. It was incumbent on the forensic scientist to provide the court with some guidance to aid them in evaluating the significance of the garbage bag correspondence.

Figure 6.4

Glad bag production process.

The general process for the manufacture of Glad Quick Tie garbage bags is diagrammed in Figure 6.4. It may seem rather complex at first blush, but the

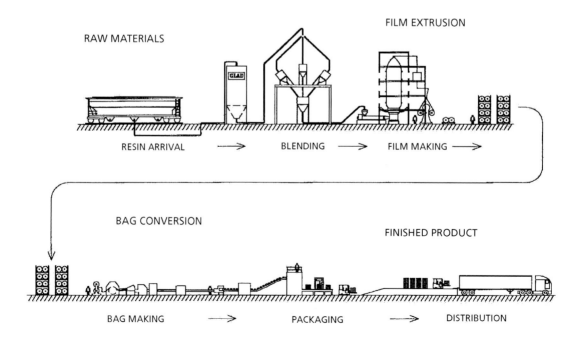

implications of understanding the process will become readily apparent in a moment. The manufacturing plant was ascertained from coding stamped on the box containing the known bags.

Virgin polyethylene resin is delivered by rail car (approximately 180,000 pounds per car) and stored in large silos (approximately two to three rail cars per silo). Other large silos hold reclaimed polyethylene acquired from the plant's internal waste; specifically, green, white, and black bags and yellow cinch drawstrings. The silos are filled from the top with resin beads and manufacture draw is taken from the bottom. The bags comprise a three-laminate co-extruded film consisting of two clear colorless outer laminates of virgin polyethylene and a thicker inner core laminate of black "master batch" and reclaimed plastic. The master batch is a blend of pigmented virgin resin pellets designed to impart the black color and opacity to the extruded film by covering up any color introduced by the reclaimed plastic. Master batch and reclaimed resin pellets are fed into blend tanks by conveyor belts, the speed of which is adjusted to change the feed (blend) rate. The output from the blend tanks is then fed to holding hoppers prior to being pneumatically fed to the line extruders. On the date of production, First Brand's Amherst, Virginia, plant ran two blown film extruders for this product (Extruder #7 and Extruder #8). There are three channels in the extrusion die permitting three-laminate co-extrusion. A separate screw extruder feeds each channel. A majority of the die lines are produced at either the die lip area or just below, where fusing of the laminates occurs. Electric eyes control the output of air blower motors, which keep the plastic "balloon" inflated to a consistent circumference. This critical function ultimately determines the height of the garbage bag. The semi-molten plastic film is constantly oscillating during the extrusion process. This, along with balloon circumference expansion and contraction (called "balloon breathing"), constantly causes slight changes in the film's die line spacing. The film can also occasionally slip at the die lips. This can result in a short-lived jump, or even reversal, in the slope of the die striae in the film. The balloon is gently guided upward five stories by wooden frames as it cools. It is then collapsed onto itself, where it runs over take-up nibs and through a hot-knife oscillating cutter which cuts two sinusoidal tie flap patterns into the center area of the collapsed (flattened) continuous film stock (Figure 6.5). The stock now consists of four separated continuous films. Two of the continuous films (A and D in Figure 6.5) have a "natural fold" at the bottom and tie flaps at the top. The remaining two continuous films (B and C in Figure 6.5) have the tie flaps running along each edge and are not folded. The B and C films run through fold-over nibs and are mechanically folded in half lengthwise to give a fold at the bottom and the tie flaps at the top. Take up nibs then split off the stock sheet and feed it onto four take-up rolls comprising the "roll set" A, B, C, and D. These rolls are now like one another, with each

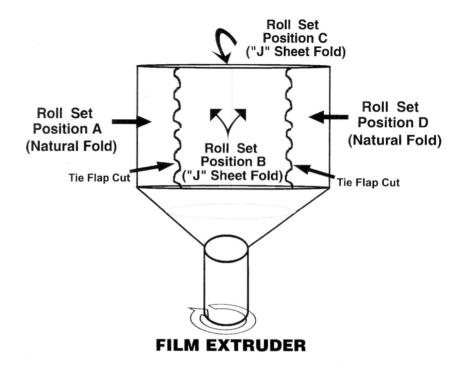

FILM EXTRUDER

consisting of a continuous film folded over onto itself with the tie flaps positioned along one side of the roll. One roll could be thought of as thousands of bags connected side by side without any side seams. The roll sets (four rolls in each set) are taken off the line approximately every two hours, weighed, and sent to an automatic roll retrieval system. The huge rolls are automatically pigeonholed in the storage rack and subsequently pulled by product type and age as needed to supply the bag machines. The stock film roll is loaded onto the front end of the bag machine. The width of the bag is controlled by the feed rate off the roll onto the machine. This rate is defined by the frequency of the sinusoidal tie flaps already cut into the stock film ("pitch"), in that there must be two flaps centered on each bag. The tie flaps are folded in onto the continuous film by a suction pad prior to the bag's sides being cut and heat-sealed. The die line extrusion machine direction, visible as striae, is now running side to side on the bags. The bag machine's cut/seal cylinder has two blades, each with both a front and back edge. This produces a seal/cut/seal function at lightning speed. Individual bags come off the line sequentially and are automatically folded and stacked into corrugated packs of 25. Each stack is pushed consecutively into a 50-count box. The process from loading the stock film roll onto the bag machine to the sealed box coming off is totally automated with no human intervention.

Bag machine speed is about 220 bags per minute, which approximates four boxes (one case) per minute. The boxes from several bag machines are pushed onto a conveyor belt that transports them to the case machine area of the plant. The boxes are diverted to the proper case machine by a bar code reader, which recognizes which product type they are. All of the 50-count boxes go to one case machine where they are boxed four to a carton (case). There may be boxes originating from several different bag machines going into one case. The cases then go to a stretch wrap unit where 52 cases are loaded onto a skid, stretch wrapped onto the skid, and fork lifted off for storage or shipment. That equates to 208 boxes of 50 bags each, or 10,400 bags per skid. The skids are then shipped to regional warehouses, where a retailer may purchase anywhere from one to 20 skids at a time.

As seen in Figure 6.5, the film stock is produced on an extrusion line that feeds four stock sheet rolls (A, B, C, and D), each weighing approximately 800 pounds. Each roll has approximately 13,000 bag equivalents on it. As previously discussed, two of the rolls have "natural folds." The tie flaps, which are located along one side of these rolls, are perfectly flush (roll set positions A and D). The other two rolls frequently have a tie flap offset resulting from a less than perfect mechanical fold-over of the two sides of the sheet following the tie flap cutting process (roll set positions B and C). They are descriptively referred to as "J sheet," with the letter "J" denoting the appearance of the offset top. Consequently, if an offset is present at the top of a quick-tie bag, it indicates the bag could only have originated from two of the four stock sheet rolls. This virtually eliminates 50 per cent of the bags produced on the extruder as having similar characteristics, as was found with the questioned and known bags in this case. As can be seen, the importance of investigating the method of production for each particular product encountered in a case cannot be overemphasized.

If one can determine the rate of rotation of the extrusion die, the number of bags produced with the characteristic predominant extrusion die pattern at any corresponding position on the bags can be determined. For example, if one full die rotation takes seven minutes there can only be two positions in that seven minutes where the striae are in the same orientation relative to the top of a bag having tie flap off-set. They would occur once at the B position and once at the C position of the roll set every full die rotation. If the manufacturer's records indicate the extrusion rate of the film is approximately 116 bag equivalents per minute, then a bag with corresponding characteristics would only be produced once every 406 bags. But for a given box of bags, how is one ever to know what the rate of rotation of the extrusion die was when those bags were produced?

If the bias (slope) of the predominant extrusion die striae pattern on the known bags in a particular case is measured (a class characteristic indicating the distance the striae systematically proceed across the bag) and the circumference of the top of the extrusion balloon is known (information available from

Figure 6.6
Extrusion die rotation
calculation.

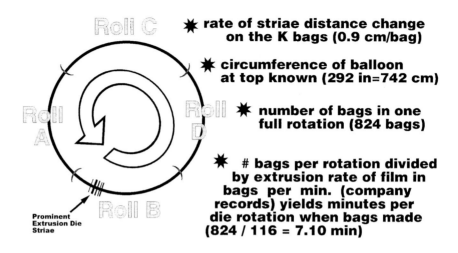

✳ **rate of striae distance change on the K bags (0.9 cm/bag)**

✳ **circumference of balloon at top known (292 in=742 cm)**

✳ **number of bags in one full rotation (824 bags)**

✳ **# bags per rotation divided by extrusion rate of film in bags per min. (company records) yields minutes per die rotation when bags made (824 / 116 = 7.10 min)**

Prominent Extrusion Die Striae

the manufacturer), one can calculate the number of bags that went through the extruder to produce one rotation of the extrusion die (Figure 6.6). If one can then ascertain the day the bags were produced (from coding on the carton of known bags) and the manufacturer keeps records of the approximate extrusion rate for film stock used on that day (in bags per minute), one can then calculate the number of minutes it took for the die to rotate one full revolution on the day the film was produced. Thus, the number of bags produced per hour having the striae in a given position relative to the top of the bags can be determined for that day. In this particular case, one such bag was produced every 3.55 minutes, half the amount of time required for one full rotation of the die. One bag would be taken up on the B stock roll and one bag taken up on the C stock roll. This equates to one such bag every 412 bags produced.

This number may not seem very unique at first impression, considering the millions of bags produced during one month. Assuming full production with no interruptions, one bag machine can produce approximately 9,500,000 bags per month. This was calculated assuming the stock rolls from both the B and C position, and the bags made from them, are indistinguishable. However, this is most likely not the case. The tie flap offset on the sheet stock, resulting from random wandering of the film during take-up on the roll, varies independently on the two rolls. These rolls may later be loaded onto two separate bag machines, which produce further variations resulting from characteristics imparted by those devices. These include bag width, centering of the tie flaps on the bag width ("wave offset" or "pitch"), and over-tuck of the tie-flaps prior to side seam sealing. If one compares sequential bags from boxes of bags produced with different rolls of stock film, corresponding "target" bags would not only have to coincide in the position of the persistent die striae, but also in the degree of tie flap offset. Both independent variables would have to correspond simultaneously, as well as the other noted characteristics imparted by the bag machines.

Consider that on one roll of stock film in the example given above, a "target" bag (one having the persistent die striae at the proper position relative to the top of the bag) will occur only 15 to 16 times in the 13,000 bag equivalents (261 boxes of 50) on the roll. The number does not sound quite so inconsequential any more. This occurs since the extruder die rotated one revolution every 7.1 minutes (2×3.55 minutes for the two time occurrence) and that one position is the only time a "target" bag will be produced on that roll. The time to produce a roll of stock film on the day the known bag's stock film was produced actually took about 110 minutes. This is known from company records of stock roll average weight, average film weight for a 50-count box of bags, and extrusion rate on the day of film production. (823 pounds average roll weight divided by 3.22 pounds average film weight per box of 50 times 50 bags per box equals approximately 12,780 bag equivalents per roll. 12,780 bag equivalents per roll divided by the 116 bags per minute average film extrusion rate equals approximately 110 minutes to produce one roll of stock film.) Thus, one "target" bag produced every 7.1 minutes of the die rotation divided into 110 minutes of production time for one stock roll equates to 16 "target" bags per roll of stock film.

The next logical question is, how long does a particular set of characteristic predominant striae remain in light of the ever changing die imperfections? Persistent striae must be used for comparison since the questioned bag was not produced consecutively to the known bags and is therefore removed some distance from them in the manufacturing process. To address this question, plant samples were acquired at approximately two-hour intervals to assess the persistence of predominant extrusion die striae patterns. This was done on two separate occasions. Two sets of samples were acquired at the First Brands Corporation Amherst plant on April 29, 1996 from one roll set position on each of the two extruders producing stock film. The third set of samples was collected over a 20-hour period on April 30 to May 1, 1997 at the same plant from one roll set position on one extruder. Ten-foot lengths of film were collected at 4.20 p.m., 5.50 p.m., 7.30 a.m., 9.25 a.m., 11.25 a.m., and 11.45 a.m.. The fourth set of samples was collected at 8.40 a.m. and 10.25 a.m. on May 1, 1997 from the other extruder in operation. All samples were taken directly from the extruder, being careful to stop the extruder die rotation at the same point every time a sample was to be taken in order to assure the same striae were being monitored. The striae patterns were inter-compared on a light box using transmitted white light. Normally, the persistent pattern was seen to change at least every two hours; however, one set of samples indicated the striae might have persisted as long as 15 hours (Figure 6.7). The initial sample was taken at the end of one day

Figure 6.7

First Brands Amherst plant sample studies.

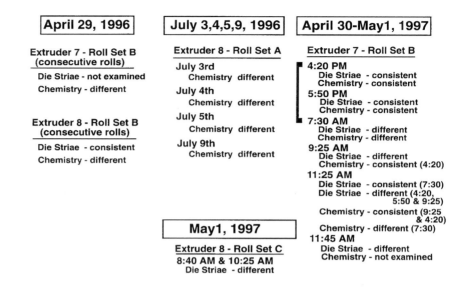

and the next sample was taken first thing the following morning. Since the change observed could have occurred at any time during that period, it was conservatively assumed that it might have changed only one minute before the second sample was taken. Taking the longest time the striae persisted, and using the calculated die rotation rate for the appropriate date the film was produced, it was determined that a maximum of approximately 254 "target" bags could have been produced on the B and C extruder roll positions with the predominant extrusion striae pattern in the position corresponding to the questioned bag. The equivalent of 16 boxes of 50 bags each would separate each "target" bag on an individual roll of stock film. On the other hand, taking the normal two-hour interval in which changes were observed, only 34 "target" bags would have been produced on two separate rolls of stock film. It is also important to recognize that even in the worst-case scenario, the resulting 254 potential "target" bags would have been spread over 16 rolls of stock film and probably loaded onto different bag machines. Unfortunately, the manufacturer's records did not permit tracking which rolls went on which bag machines. It is, however, unlikely that all of these bags would have corresponding construction characteristics, as discussed earlier. The evidential significance of such a limited number of bags corresponding to the questioned bag's physical characteristics when contrasted to the millions produced is quite striking.

Both Kopec and Meyers (1980) and Nir-El (1994) have discussed the value of not only studying physical characteristics in plastic bag comparisons, but also chemical characteristics. As mentioned earlier, the plastic sheet comprising the Glad Garbage Bags with Quick Tie Flaps is of a three-laminate construction.

The outer laminates are virgin non-pigmented polyethylene, while the thicker center laminate is composed primarily of internal waste polyethylene. The plastic waste comes from various products produced in the plant, including white, black, and green trash bags along with yellow cinch ties. The proportion of colors stored in the reclaimed plastic silo is neither controlled nor monitored and consequently the concentration of pigments present in the reclaimed plastic varies randomly. Titanium dioxide (white) and yellow iron oxide (used to produce the green product line) proved to vary the most.

X-ray fluorescence spectroscopic analysis (XRF) was conducted on two 25 mm by 25 mm square samples of individual bags. The samples were taken from one side of the plastic bag/film and introduced to the instrument as ethanol-wiped single-layer films (including all three laminates) stretched over a plastic aperture. Each sample was analyzed twice, originally and then again after rotating the specimen 90 degrees. Spectra were collected on a Phillips/EDAX PV9500 energy-dispersive XRF spectrometer using a 40 KV x-ray beam emitted from a rhodium x-ray tube operated at a 500 micro-ampere beam current for approximately 3500 live seconds at a 20 per cent dead-time. The tube was fitted with a 7 mm diameter steel collimator to control sampling area. The background was subtracted from the resultant spectra, peak identifications made and peak intensities acquired. The resultant peak intensities for magnesium (Mg), aluminum (Al), silicon (Si), phosphorous (P), sulfur (S), potassium (K), calcium (Ca), titanium (Ti), chromium (Cr), iron (Fe), copper (Cu), and zinc (Zn) K-alpha lines as well as for the lead (Pb) L-alpha lines were then ratioed to the rhodium (Rh) L-alpha tube scatter peak. The mean, standard deviation, and relative standard deviation for these ratios were then calculated for the four runs.

In order to evaluate the variation of elemental constituents in the bag film, the same samples acquired at First Brands Corporation's Amherst plant for studying die striae persistence were analyzed by XRF. These plant samples concentrated on variations that might occur within a one-day period. Plant samples taken from one roll set position on one extruder at the Amherst plant on 3, 4, 5 and July 9, 1996, and a box of bags purchased at a local Albertson's grocery store and manufactured at the Amherst plant on January 6, 1996 were also acquired and analyzed. Results from samples taken on different days (Table 6.1) and even within one day (Table 6.2) demonstrate a variation in the titanium and/or iron elemental concentrations observed by XRF. Of course, these random elemental variations are not as discriminating as the die striae pattern variations, considering that they will be found in all bags produced in that time frame and are more likely to repeat themselves inadvertently over time. Nonetheless, they do vary over relatively short periods of time totally independent of other comparison characteristics.

Sample	Ti ratio to Rh ($\times$ 100)			Fe ratio to Rh ($\times$ 100)		
	Mean	SD	Rel. SD (%)	Mean	SD	Rel. SD (%)
Box of 50 from store 01/06/96						
Albertson's Box – Bag 1	35.4	1.1	3.0	42.0	1.4	3.4
Albertson's Box – Bag 2	34.4	0.8	2.3	39.2	0.8	2.1
First Brands plant samples 04/29/96						
Successive rolls – Tower 7						
Roll 1	71.0	1.1	0.1	5.4	0.2	4.0
Roll 2	60.3	0.9	1.5	5.0	0.5	9.7
Successive rolls – Tower 8						
Roll 1	70.4	2.8	3.9	5.0	0.2	4.5
Roll 2	60.7	1.8	2.9	5.8	0.1	2.1
First Brands plant samples						
Roll set position A						
Line 8 – Day 1 (7/3/96)	6.6	0.4	5.7	4.0	0.2	5.9
Line 8 – Day 2 (7/4/96)	7.1	0.2	2.7	12.4	0.7	5.3
Line 8 – Day 3 (7/5/96)	17.7	0.1	0.6	2.7	0.1	1.4
Line 8 – Day 7 (7/9/96)	18.3	0.3	1.9	6.5	0.3	4.1
Roll set position C						
Line 8 – Day 2 (7/4/96)	7.4	0.2	2.7	12.7	0.2	1.7
First Brands plant samples						
Line 7 – Roll B						
4/30/97, 4.20 p.m.	94.7	1.5	1.6	8.8	0.6	6.4
4/30/97, 5.50 p.m.	98.9	6.1	6.2	9.7	0.8	8.3
5/01/97, 7.30 a.m.	84.2	2.9	3.4	8.1	0.1	1.5
5/01/97, 9.25 a.m.	89.4	1.6	1.8	8.4	0.2	2.1
5/01/97, 11.25 a.m.	91.7	2.5	2.7	8.6	0.3	3.0

Table 6.1

Titanium and iron ratios on Amherst plant samples over time.

Table 6.2 (opposite)

Elemental ratios on Amherst plant: samples over 19 hours.

In order for a given bag to have originated from a box of bags, the persistent die striae, the elemental ratios, and the tie flap offset must all correspond to the bags remaining in the box. Additionally, this offset varies sequentially even within a box of bags, and the questioned bag's offset measurement should coincide with the offset sequence pattern of the bags remaining in the box. All of these criteria were met when comparing the bag found on Jenny's body with the box of bags discovered in the defendant's apartment.

INTERPRETATION

Visual examination and comparison of the garbage bag recovered from Jenny Kilborn's body with the one loose bag and the bags remaining in the box of Glad Quick-Tie 30-gallon garbage bags discovered in the defendant's apartment revealed corresponding construction characteristics and predominant die striae indicating the bags were produced by the same manufacturer, in the same plant, on the same extrusion line, and in approximately the same time frame.

Further comparison of the position of the predominant die striae relative to

Sample	Mg	Al	Si	P	S	K	Ca	Ti	Cr	Fe	Zn	Pb	Rh
Line 7 – Roll position B	(XRF peak intensity ratios normalized to Rh peak area)												
4/30/97 4.20 p.m. Sam.1A	0.01	0.01	0.21	0.05	0.22	0.02	0.01	0.95	0.01	0.08	0.03	0.01	1.00
4/30/97 4.20 p.m. Sam.1B	0.01	0.01	0.20	0.04	0.22	0.01	0.01	0.92	0.01	0.09	0.03	0.01	1.00
4/30/97 4.20 p.m. Sam. 2A	0.01	0.01	0.20	0.04	0.22	0.01	0.01	0.96	0.00	0.09	0.03	0.01	1.00
4/30/97 4.20 p.m. Sam. 2B	0.01	0.01	0.17	0.04	0.23	0.01	0.01	0.96	0.00	0.09	0.03	0.01	1.00
Mean	**0.01**	**0.01**	**0.20**	**0.04**	**0.23**	**0.01**	**0.01**	**0.95**	**0.00**	**0.09**	**0.03**	**0.01**	**1.00**
Standard deviation (SD)	**0.00**	**0.00**	**0.01**	**0.00**	**0.00**	**0.00**	**0.00**	**0.02**	**0.00**	**0.01**	**0.00**	**0.00**	**0.00**
Relative SD (RSD)	**12.67**	**7.10**	**6.44**	**5.82**	**2.11**	**28.19**	**33.15**	**1.63**	**55.81**	**6.41**	**2.53**	**18.24**	**0.00**
4/30/97 5.50 p.m. Sam.1A	0.01	0.01	0.20	0.05	0.24	0.01	0.01	0.94	0.00	0.09	0.03	0.01	1.00
4/30/97 5.50 p.m. Sam.1B	0.01	0.01	0.19	0.04	0.24	0.01	0.01	0.92	0.00	0.09	0.02	0.01	1.00
4/30/97 5.50 p.m. Sam. 2A	0.01	0.01	0.19	0.05	0.25	0.02	0.01	1.05	0.00	0.11	0.03	0.01	1.00
4/30/97 5.50 p.m. Sam. 2B	0.01	0.01	0.17	0.04	0.25	0.02	0.01	1.04	0.00	0.10	0.03	0.01	1.00
Mean	**0.01**	**0.01**	**0.19**	**0.04**	**0.25**	**0.01**	**0.01**	**0.99**	**0.00**	**0.10**	**0.03**	**0.01**	**1.00**
SD	**0.00**	**0.00**	**0.01**	**0.00**	**0.01**	**0.00**	**0.00**	**0.06**	**0.00**	**0.01**	**0.00**	**0.00**	**0.00**
RSD	**17.72**	**9.86**	**5.93**	**5.48**	**2.30**	**25.41**	**24.72**	**6.16**	**26.73**	**8.32**	**10.64**	**17.80**	**0.00**
5/1/97 7.30 a.m. Sam.1A	0.01	0.01	0.21	0.05	0.19	0.02	0.01	0.83	0.00	0.08	0.03	0.01	1.00
5/1/97 7.30 a.m. Sam.1B	0.01	0.01	0.19	0.04	0.19	0.01	0.01	0.81	0.00	0.08	0.03	0.01	1.00
5/1/97 7.30 a.m. Sam. 2A	0.01	0.01	0.19	0.05	0.20	0.01	0.01	0.89	0.00	0.08	0.03	0.01	1.00
5/1/97 7.30 a.m. Sam. 2B	0.01	0.01	0.21	0.05	0.20	0.02	0.02	0.83	0.01	0.08	0.03	0.01	1.00
Mean	**0.01**	**0.01**	**0.20**	**0.05**	**0.19**	**0.02**	**0.01**	**0.84**	**0.00**	**0.08**	**0.03**	**0.01**	**1.00**
SD	**0.00**	**0.00**	**0.01**	**0.00**	**0.01**	**0.00**	**0.00**	**0.03**	**0.00**	**0.00**	**0.00**	**0.00**	**0.00**
RSD	**16.17**	**8.60**	**4.72**	**7.21**	**2.93**	**28.53**	**9.68**	**3.43**	**41.02**	**1.52**	**2.67**	**23.08**	**0.00**
5/1/97 9.25 a.m. Sam.1A	0.01	0.01	0.22	0.05	0.23	0.02	0.01	0.88	0.01	0.09	0.03	0.01	1.00
5/1/97 9.25 a.m. Sam.1B	0.01	0.01	0.22	0.04	0.23	0.01	0.01	0.87	0.00	0.08	0.03	0.01	1.00
5/1/97 9.25 a.m. Sam. 2A	0.01	0.01	0.22	0.04	0.24	0.01	0.02	0.90	0.00	0.09	0.02	0.01	1.00
5/1/97 9.25 a.m. Sam. 2B	0.01	0.01	0.22	0.04	0.25	0.01	0.01	0.91	0.00	0.09	0.03	0.01	1.00
Mean	**0.01**	**0.01**	**0.22**	**0.04**	**0.24**	**0.01**	**0.01**	**0.89**	**0.00**	**0.08**	**0.03**	**0.01**	**1.00**
SD	**0.00**	**0.00**	**0.00**	**0.00**	**0.01**	**0.00**	**0.00**	**0.02**	**0.00**	**0.00**	**0.00**	**0.00**	**0.00**
RSD	**14.18**	**6.67**	**0.89**	**6.94**	**2.61**	**31.21**	**15.18**	**1.82**	**39.97**	**2.06**	**7.66**	**13.47**	**0.00**
5/1/97 11.25 a.m. Sam.1A	0.01	0.01	0.21	0.05	0.21	0.01	0.01	0.92	0.00	0.09	0.03	0.01	1.00
5/1/97 11.25 a.m. Sam.1B	0.01	0.01	0.20	0.04	0.21	0.01	0.01	0.88	0.00	0.08	0.03	0.01	1.00
5/1/97 11.25 a.m. Sam. 2A	0.01	0.01	0.21	0.05	0.22	0.02	0.01	0.92	0.00	0.09	0.03	0.01	1.00
5/1/97 11.25 a.m. Sam. 2B	0.01	0.01	0.20	0.05	0.22	0.01	0.02	0.95	0.00	0.09	0.03	0.01	1.00
Mean	**0.01**	**0.01**	**0.21**	**0.04**	**0.22**	**0.01**	**0.01**	**0.92**	**0.00**	**0.09**	**0.03**	**0.01**	**1.00**
SD	**0.00**	**0.00**	**0.00**	**0.00**	**0.01**	**0.00**	**0.00**	**0.02**	**0.00**	**0.00**	**0.00**	**0.00**	**0.00**
RSD	**10.31**	**4.07**	**2.36**	**7.69**	**2.87**	**32.02**	**29.05**	**2.70**	**10.97**	**3.00**	**3.01**	**27.77**	**0.00**

the top of the bags between the bag recovered from Jenny's body and the loose bag in the defendant's apartment indicate the questioned bag was removed in production only one to two bags from the loose bag in the apartment, if it did indeed originate from the same box of bags. Similar examinations showed the loose bag in the apartment was manufactured two bags after the 16 bags remaining in the box of Glad Quick-Tie 30-gallon garbage bags found in the defendant's apartment, under the caveat that it is reasonable to assume that the loose bag found in the apartment did originate from the same box of bags as that discovered in the apartment.

A study of bags purchased at a local retail store and acquired directly from the manufacturer of the case bags indicates that extrusion die striae persistence and chemistry vary independent of one another, but may be stable for up to 15 hours on a given extruder. This is not apparently the norm, however, considering that at least five of the seven successive stock roll samples acquired from the manufacturer (equating to approximately two hours of extruder run time) were differentiated either by variations in extrusion die striae or differences in their elemental (chemical) profiles. These stock rolls are subsequently placed on independent bag machines, where other differing characteristics are imparted to the bags within a box, such as width, centering of the tie flaps on the bag width, and over-tuck of the tie-flaps. Furthermore, the tie flap offset on the B and C rolls of film stock from a stock roll set varies independently on the two rolls as a result of random wandering of the film during take-up on the roll. For a questioned bag to correspond to an existing partially used box of bags, all independent characteristics would have to simultaneously coincide. That includes persistent die striae, elemental chemical characteristics, tie flap offsets, bag widths, degree of tie-flap centering, and either the lack or presence of tie-flap over-tucks. It is unlikely that bags produced from numerous rolls of stock film would correspond in all of these characteristics.

Considering the information developed from the plant visit and plant sample studies, two reasonable scenarios were developed to evaluate the number of boxes of bags produced potentially containing "target" bags like the one found on Jenny's body. The first was most favorable to the defense, based on the most conservative evaluation of the information accumulated. It included all bags which would have been produced having the characteristic striae in the proper position relative to the top of the bag from rolls of stock film taken from both the B and C position of the roll sets produced over a 15-hour period. It took into account neither independent construction variations imparted to separate stock rolls (tie flap offset wandering) nor independent variations imparted by different bag machines. Sixteen "target" bags on each of 16 stock rolls would yield 256 "target" bags in existence. The target bags would be found one per box, resulting in only 256 boxes containing a target bag. Between each of these boxes, there are 16 boxes containing no target bag. Considering there are 208 boxes per skid, the target bags would thus be spread over approximately 20 skids. Manufacturer records indicate that it would not be unreasonable to assume that all 20 skids were shipped to one distribution warehouse, where they would then have been sold to retailers covering three-quarters of the state of Florida and all of Puerto Rico.

The second scenario was most favorable to the prosecution, based on the more realistic evaluation of the information acquired. A two-hour period with no change in characteristics would result in just over one roll set being produced. This would result in 17 "target" bags being produced on stock rolls in the B roll set position and 17 "target" bags being produced on stock rolls in the C roll set position. Due to natural folds and subsequently no tie flap offset at the top of the bags, the A and D roll set positions can be excluded as potential sources. Again, assuming no differences resulting from independent variations imparted to separate stock rolls (tie flap offset wandering) nor independent variations imparted by different bag machines, this would result in only 34 "target" bags in existence. They would be spread over three to six skids of bags packaged for shipment and would most likely be shipped to the same distribution warehouse. Of course, even this scenario makes some strong assumptions. It assumes that the two stock rolls were loaded on the same bag machine. If they had been loaded on two separate bag machines, it would have been unusual for the resulting bags to be like one another in their construction characteristics. This is possible, but unusual. It also assumes that the two stock rolls have similar tie flap offset characteristics. Again, this is possible, but unusual. Instead, it is more reasonable to suspect the number of boxes having "target" bags in them to be well below the projected 34.

And finally, in both these scenarios, one must consider that the sequence of the "target" bag in each of the potential source boxes must be such that it simultaneously coincides with the pattern of change in the tie flap offset within the box of 50 bags. Furthermore, one must recognize that some of the potential source boxes, whether it be 256 or 34, were either not opened or still had the "target" bag in them at the time of this investigation. And of course, these boxes could not have been potential sources for the bag found on Jenny's body, unlike the box of bags found in John Cameron's apartment where the "target" bag was only one to two bags removed in sequence from the remaining bags.

SUMMARY

This investigation served to illustrate once again the value of class evidence in building a circumstantial evidence case, especially in the absence of other individualizing evidence, such as multiple probe DNA and latent fingerprints.

Without it, the case would have been on a charted course for failure. It also brings with it a glimpse at some of the potential complications in the interpretation of classical trace evidence, including hair and fiber transfers. Known prior contact between the sources of transferred material severely handicaps any attempt to associate the subject or victim based on the presence of contact trace. Evidential significance in this case would hinge upon arguments against transfer by casual contact considering the quantity of dog hair transferred as well as for the presence of transferred fibers on the victim's skin, which would normally not retain fibers for an extended period of time.

After a Frye hearing, the voiceprint analysis results were accepted by the court as reliable evidence that could be introduced during trial. Expert testimony placed an 80 per cent confidence level on association of the voice in the 911 call with that of the defendant.

The garbage bag examination stresses the importance of thoroughly investigating and understanding the method of production for any product being examined, if the forensic scientist hopes to maximize evidential significance. The background knowledge acquired permitted testimony beyond the constraints of "originated from the same manufacturer, the same plant, the same extrusion line and in approximately the same time frame." It gave the court a defendable estimate of what the phrase "same time frame" means and generated an understanding of the magnitude of the number of other potential boxes of bags which could have been a source of the bag found on Jenny Kilborn's body. The number was surprisingly small, even in the most favorable assessment for the defense. The testimony proffered withstood hours of pretrial depositions along with a Frye hearing, where it was accepted as viable evidence.

The mitochondrial DNA hair evidence was excluded following a Frye hearing, surprisingly declared by the presiding judge as too novel a technique at this time in the State of Florida. Yet, from the bench, the same judge referred to the plastic bag evidence as "very compelling." As can be seen, and is known by all that enter it, the legal arena is filled with surprises. Although distastefully time consuming from a management viewpoint, the potential legal impact of fully developing arguments for class evidence significance can never be underestimated.

And in that same legal arena, fraught with surprises and hardly designed for work product efficiency, yet another surprise turn of events unfolded. John Cameron pleaded guilty to second degree murder one week after the Frye hearing on the plastic bag examination and is currently serving a forty-year sentence without the possibility of parole. Perhaps this brings some peace of mind for dear little Jenny and those who loved her.

ACKNOWLEDGEMENTS

I would like to thank First Brands Corporation for its full support during this investigation. The time, knowledge, and ingenuity of Mr Noel Roberts, Senior Quality Engineer, permitted much of the background information to be developed and collected. First Brands Corporation's commitment to quality assurance procedures provided much of the documentation necessary in reconstructing the manufacturing process of the plastic bags. My further appreciation to Mr Dave Zirnsak, plant manager of First Brands Corporation's Amherst, Virginia plant. He and his staff did all they could to help both the prosecuting attorney and me understand the manufacturing process and witness it firsthand. I would also like to thank my colleagues, Ms Marianne Hildreth, Ms Jan Taylor, and Ms Marta Strawser, for reviewing my work on the case and this chapter. As with every day, their skills, insight, and questions helped to fill in voids and address the inadequacies. And finally, a word of appreciation to Mr Christopher White, Assistant State Attorney for the Eighteenth Judicial Circuit for the State of Florida. Every once in a while, in every forensic scientist's career, I hope they have the opportunity to work with such a dedicated and skilled attorney – one who takes interest in the expert's work and makes a genuine effort to understand it. The effort on the attorney's part, as demonstrated in this case, is well rewarded by enabling him to provide effective communication between the expert witness and the court. The results speak for themselves.

REFERENCES

Castle, D.A., Gibbins, B., and Hamer, P.S. (1994) *J. For. Sci. Soc.*, 34(1), 61–68.

Kidd, C.B.M. and Robertson, J. (1982) *J. For. Sci. Soc.*, 22, 301–308.

Kopec, R.J. and Meyers, C.R. (1980). *AFTE Journal*, 12(1), 23–26.

Locard, E. (1928) *Police J.*, 1(2), 177–192.

Locard, E. (1930) *Am. J. Police Sci.*, 1(3), 276–298; 1(4), 401–418; 1(5), 496–514.

Nir-El, Y. (1994). *J. For. Sci.*, 39(3), 758–768.

Pounds, C.A. and Smalldon, K.W. (1975) *J. For. Sci. Soc.*, 15, 197–207.

Robertson, J., Kidd, C.B.M., and Parkinson, H.M.P. (1982) *J. For. Sci. Soc.*, 22, 353–360.

Stanko, R.F., and Attenberger, D.W. (1996) *CAC Newsletter*, Fall, 14–15.

Von Bremen, U.G. and Blunt, L.K.R. (1983) *J. For. Sci.*, 28(3), 644–654.

CHAPTER 7

MANSLAUGHTER CAUSED BY A HIT-AND-RUN: GLASS AS EVIDENCE OF ASSOCIATION

José R. Almirall

INTRODUCTION

A great many advances in analytical chemistry have improved the characterizations of the organic and inorganic components in the small fragments of materials that are often encountered in scenes of crime due to contact transfers. The scientific review and standardization of these sensitive techniques by forensic scientists aids the judiciary in accepting these analytical methods as admissible and relevant to legal proceedings where physical evidence is considered. The challenge to forensic scientists who are interpreting materials analysis is to express their opinion without understating or overstating the value of the evidence under consideration. The presentation of a case I was involved with while working for the Miami-Dade Police Department (MDPD) Crime Laboratory Bureau is helpful to appreciate the value of small amounts of transfer evidence. This case is especially significant to trace evidence examiners – the chemists and physical scientists who examine materials to determine if an association exists between a sample recovered at a crime scene and a source linking the perpetrator. While advances in molecular biology and the advent of "DNA fingerprinting" techniques have truly revolutionized forensic science since the late 1980s in the US, these methods could not be employed in this case nor can they be employed in many similar cases involving the transfer of materials. Another reason for mentioning the case is that it exemplifies the recklessness and foolishness of someone leaving the scene of an accident. A tragic death may have been prevented in this case had the perpetrator stopped after the accident and attempted to provide medical attention to the victim. His decision to leave the scene changed an automobile accident into a felony hit-and-run.

The violent nature of vehicle accidents, even at slow speeds, produces a variety of transfer evidence making it *impossible* for the perpetrator to leave the scene "without a trace". It is this physical evidence that trace examiners evaluate to determine whether an association between the perpetrator and the crime scene is likely or, in some cases, certain.

THE CRIME SCENE

On Saturday, June 24, 1995 at 5.50 a.m., a witness called the Providenciales police station to report that she had seen the body of a female on the side of the road near Leeward Highway in Providenciales, the most populated of the Turks and Caicos islands. The Turks and Caicos is a group of 30 islands in the Caribbean located southeast of the Bahamas Islands. Its government is designated as a British overseas territory with a legal system based on the laws of England and Wales, a total population of 17,502 and a total area approximately 2.5 times the size of Washington DC.

The victim, a 42-year-old female Dominican national, was walking home shortly after midnight, at the end of her shift from her job as a waitress when she was apparently struck by a vehicle. Her body was found face down about nine feet from the paved road. She was dressed in a black T-shirt and blue jeans. The doctor who pronounced her dead at the scene noted that she had two lacerations to the right side of her head, abrasions to the side of her chest and small bruises on her hands and upper body. A local constable who had received training in crime scene processing in Miami, FL, was summoned to the scene and began documenting the area surrounding the body. A summary of his report listed the following items found: earrings, a watch, a pendant and chain, eyeglasses, a headband, debris appearing to be undercoating from a vehicle, and nine large glass fragments scattered around the body appearing to come from a vehicle headlamp. The constable photographed the items in their original position, measured the distances from the body, packaged and sealed the items after assigning them unique evidence identifiers. He also collected control samples of soil in the areas surrounding the body.

A possible suspect was identified 11 days later on July 5 when he was visited by the constable to inquire about the incident. The suspect denied being involved with the accident and requested the presence of his attorney during the interview. A preliminary examination of the vehicle indicated considerable damage to the top and side of the left (driver's side) front fender just over the left wheel. Also noted was damage to the bumper on the same side and one of the headlamps on that side was missing (this older model vehicle has two headlamps on each side, one right above the other). The car was then moved to a shop for further processing. Careful examination of the damaged area did not yield any type of biological evidence such as blood, skin or hair. Apparently, the vehicle had been washed and cleaned thoroughly in the previous days. The constable did find fragments of broken glass lodged in the bumper and inside the lamp assembly of the missing lamp. The intact lamp above the missing lamp was collected and also packaged. Standard paint samples were collected along with a standard sample of debris from the underside of the vehicle. The vehicle was photographed (see Figures 7.1 and 7.2) and impounded by the police.

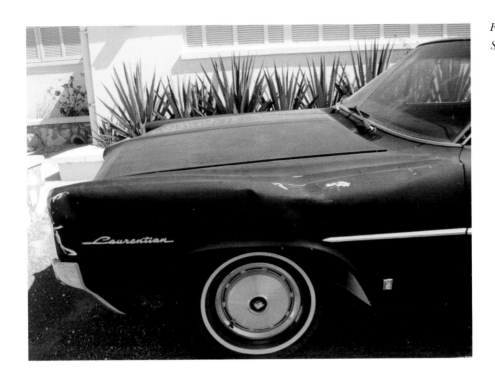

Figure 7.1
Side view of damage area.

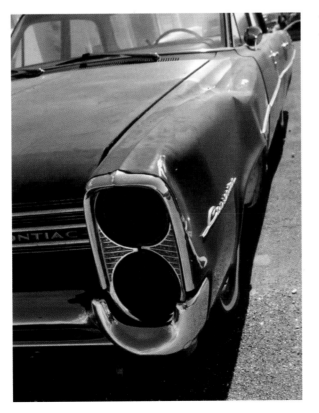

Figure 7.2
Front view of damage.

ANALYSIS

On August 10, 1995, the Miami-Dade Police Crime Laboratory received several packages of evidence along with a list of items contained in the labeled and sealed bags. The analysis request form included instructions for the examiner to determine if there was an association between the glass fragments found at the scene and the broken glass pieces found on the vehicle belonging to the suspect.

The Miami-Dade laboratory is equipped to measure the density and refractive index of forensic sized fragments and collaborates with the Departments of Chemistry and Geology of Florida International University in Miami, FL to use the university instrumentation to measure the elemental composition in small glass fragments.

The first step in any glass comparison is to inspect the fragments visually and determine if there exists a fracture match between any of the recovered fragments to any of the source fragments. Although very rarely found, such a match would positively link the fragments as originating from the same source. No match was found in this case. The condition of the recovered fragments is also of interest and, in this case, examination revealed that the fragments were clean and without scratch markings, indicating a relatively recent transfer of the glass to the scene (environmental elements and scene conditions change the appearance of glass over time allowing for old glass to be distinguished from "fresh" glass). The number of fragments found (nine) and their size was also of probative interest. Some of the recovered fragments also had markings imparted during the manufacturing process including the number 2 and the letters "e-a-l-e-d" with a missing piece in front of the letters and the letters "G-U" in a square (see Figures 7.3 and 7.4) with the remainder of the letters missing. These markings are similar to those found on vehicle sealed beam headlamps.

Figures 7.3 and 7.4

Glass fragments recovered from the crime scene. Markings suggest these fragments originate from a vehicle headlamp.

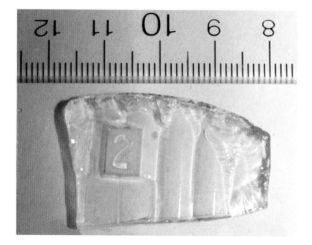
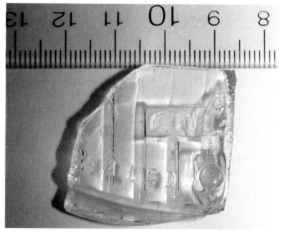

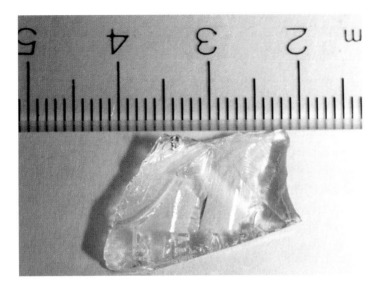

Figure 7.5

Glass fragments removed from the vehicle. Markings suggest the letters BE and a partial A.

The intact headlamp removed from the vehicle had a number "1" at the top of the lamp, the word "Guide" in a square and the words "Sealed Beam" at the bottom. A glass fragment removed from the vehicle had the letters "B-E" and a portion of a letter "A" (see Figure 7.5) with the remainder missing.

After photography, samples from the nine fragments found at the scene were compared to 10 fragments found on the vehicle by refractive index (RI) measurements. The fragments from the vehicle would be treated as originating from one source and grouped together to calculate a mean RI value and compared to each of the recovered fragments. In most glass comparisons, thickness measurements are taken and compared. Thickness measurements in this case would not provide comparative information, as is also the case with most container glass comparisons. Headlamps and containers are manufactured in molds, producing uneven and heterogeneous thickness throughout the entire unit. Thickness comparisons are reserved for glass thought to originate from flat glass such as windows where the thickness is expected to be homogeneous throughout the entire window.

Due to the high correlation between RI and density, little (if any) information is gained by density measurements if RI is measured. Indices of refraction are now easily and quickly determined and provide numerical data to compare one group of fragments to other fragments. The MDPD protocol also calls for elemental composition analysis to be performed if the RI does not distinguish the source from the recovered fragments. In this case, density measurements were not performed but refractive index measurements were compared between the recovered fragments and fragments found on the vehicle.

REFRACTIVE INDEX MEASUREMENTS

BACKGROUND

Refractive index comparisons can provide a good measure of discrimination between glasses of different origins. Crime laboratories have been employing the optical properties of glass to distinguish between fragments for over 60 years and RI is currently the primary method of glass analysis in crime laboratories. A thorough treatment of the theory and application of RI measurements can be found in a recent publication by Almirall *et al.* (2000).

Refractive Index is a measure of the change of direction (refraction) that is observed when light passes from one medium to another. Refraction can be described as the interaction between the light and a transparent medium where V_{vacuum} is the velocity of light in a vacuum (or air, for practical purposes) and V_{glass} is the velocity of light in the transparent glass. Since the velocity will always be greater in a vacuum, Equation 7.1 describes this ratio as always equal to or greater than 1. The more refractive materials such as diamond (~2.42) or leaded glass (~1.55) have greater RI values than soda-lime window glass (~1.52) or borosilicate headlamp glass (~1.48).

$$\mathrm{RI} = \frac{V_{vacuum}}{V_{glass}} \tag{7.1}$$

The first refractive index measurements of glass were accomplished by observing bright lines moving into and out of the glass from surrounding oil while defocusing the glass. These moving lines were first described by Becké (1892) while observing geological samples and later applied to glass. To measure RI, the glass is immersed in oil and the focus is adjusted on the edge of the glass fragment. When the objective is raised, if the bright line moves into the oil, it indicates that the oil has a higher RI than the glass. A miscible liquid can be added to the oil to lower the RI until the line does not move further or disappears. At that point, the RI of the oil is equal to the RI of the glass and the RI of the oil can be measured with a refractometer. Emmons later described the temperature variation method observing that RI varied with temperature. As the temperature of oil is increased, the RI of the oil decreases while not affecting the RI of the immersed glass to the same extent.

The advent of the Mettler hot stage in the early 1970s improved the control of the temperature of the slide thereby improving on the accuracy and precision of the measurements. The double variation method incorporates the variation of both the temperature of the oil and the wavelength of the light coming through the sample to determine the RI for three wavelengths. The Association of Analytical Chemists (1990) published the double variation method as a standard method of analysis.

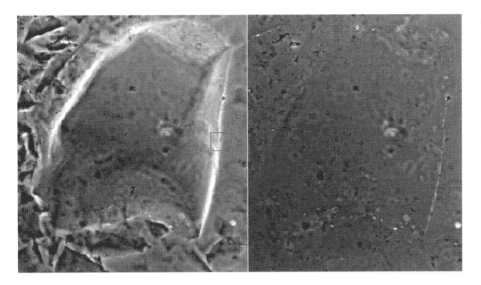

In the mid 1980s, Foster and Freeman developed an instrument that they called Glass Refractive Index Measurement (GRIM) based on the coupling of a computer-controlled Mettler hot stage, a phase contrast microscope and the oil immersion technique (see Figure 7.6 for contrast views).

The American Society of Testing and Materials has recently published a standard test method for the determination of RI of glass samples using the oil immersion method and a phase contrast microscope (ASTM 2000). The method reports that a standard deviation (SD) of 0.00002 can be expected for the operation of the instrument over a five-hour period and an SD of 0.00003 can be expected over a five-day period.

Three studies have been conducted (Locke 1985; Collins and Kobus 1987; Cassista and Sandercock 1994) to evaluate the accuracy, precision and long-term stability of the GRIM method. These extensive evaluations of the GRIM in the UK, Canada and Australia conclude that the instrument provides for very satisfactory results and should be the method of choice for the measurement of RI in forensic laboratories.

REFRACTIVE INDEX MEASUREMENTS OF HEADLAMP GLASSES

Ojena and De Forest (1972) reported on the variation of RI within a single headlamp and between lamps manufactured at the same plant over a three-month period based on a study conducted in 1972. These authors report a relatively large variation within a single lamp, especially within a single reflector and they attribute the large variation to thermal effects during the manufacturing and molding process as well as possible heterogeneity in the glass melt. The reported range of RI for the four brands sampled at 18 locations were 0.00026,

0.00009, 0.00018, and 0.00048 for the lenses and 0.00076, 0.00033, 0.00054 and 0.00112 for the reflectors. A total of 296 glass specimens were also collected over a three-month period from three manufacturers, Corning, Anchor-Hocking and General Electric, and the lamps exhibited a variation of 0.00124, 0.00070 and 0.00041 respectively over that time. They also conducted an automobile wrecking-yard study, taking multiple measurements of 24 headlamps. The overall range for all the lamps examined was 0.00363. The authors also report the average standard deviation (0.000034) for the measurement was less than the expected variation across a single lamp.

In 1993, 73 automobile headlamps removed from a wide variety of automobiles, including European and Japanese manufacturers, representing more than 20 years of manufacturing dates were collected from a wrecking yard in Dade County, FL in a study by the author(Almirall *et al.* 1996).

A single headlamp lens and a single reflector were sampled across the unit in nine different locations. The range for the lens was found to be 0.00020 with a SD of 0.00006. The results for the reflector were similar. The overall range for all the lamps examined was 0.00340 (1.47604–1.47944). Nineteen (19) two standard deviation (2 SD) wide bins were constructed to describe the data (see Figure 7.7) for all the headlamps in the Dade study. Fifteen of the bins were populated and the most populated RI bin (1.47894) had a frequency of 11 samples. As in the Ojena study, the overall range was found to be relatively small in comparison with the overall ranges found for a similar evaluation of containers (overall variation of 0.02615 for 146 containers collected in Florida over a

Figure 7.7

RI distribution for 73 headlamps from a wrecking yard.

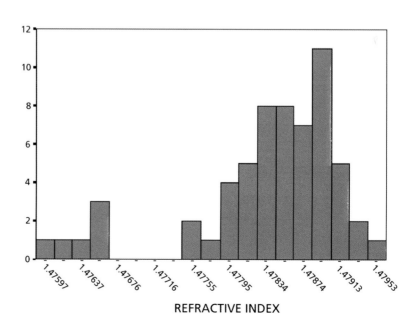

REFRACTIVE INDEX

three-year period) and sheet glasses (overall variation of 0.01313 for 465 sheet glass samples collected over a period of three years). Additionally, the variation within a single unit for headlamps is quite large in comparison with single unit variations for containers or sheet glass. This combination of factors results in poor discrimination power of RI comparisons for headlamps, as illustrated by the low number of "bins" in Figure 7.7.

Another way of evaluating the discrimination power of the measurement is to conduct a pairwise comparison of the 73 headlamps examined.

There are $n(n-1)/2$ ways to compare n sample means with each other while excluding the comparison of the sample mean with itself. The Dade database includes 60 of the headlamp samples for 1770 possible comparisons. Tukey's HSD test was used in a post-hoc test of a one-way Analysis of Variance (ANOVA) of the data to evaluate all of the pairwise comparisons (Johnson and Wichern 1992). Approximately 37 per cent, that is 654 of the 1770 possible pairs of all headlamps *cannot* be distinguished from each other even though all 60 lamps originated from different sources. The results of the Ojena and Dade studies indicate that RI comparisons of headlamps provide limited informing power as to the value of a "match" between fragments.

METHODOLOGY

The Miami-Dade Police Department is equipped with a GRIM2 for RI measurements. The instrument was calibrated and operated as described in the method ASTM E1967 at a single wavelength (sodium D line, 589.3 nm) (ASTM 2000). Locke glass standards and immersion oils were used for the RI determinations and to calibrate the instrument. The refractive index values were reported at the match temperature.

CASE RESULTS

Ten of the fragments that were found on the suspect's vehicle were selected at random from the large number of fragments submitted. The RI of each of the fragments was measured and found to range from 1.47762–1.47784, a mean of 1.47773 and a SD of 0.00008. Each of nine (9) fragments found on the side of the road at the accident scene were also measured for RI. The values obtained were: 1.47771, 1.47771, 1.47772, 1.47774, 1.47775, 1.47777, 1.47777, 1.47782, 1.47782. All nine fragments met the match criteria when comparing to the mean ± 2 SD and therefore were analytically indistinguishable from the mean of the standards. Given the data presented above about the weakness of RI to differentiate between headlamps, written reports and testimony should be worded such that the value of a "match" by RI is not overstated.

As a matter of policy, the MDPD laboratory performs elemental analysis on those cases where the RI does not distinguish between the samples.

ELEMENTAL ANALYSIS

BACKGROUND

Elemental analysis of glass specimens is a useful classification tool to determine if glass originates from containers, sheet, and borosilicate glass sources such as headlamps or cooking ware. Table 7.1 is a list of the typical elemental concentrations for the major and minor components in float, container, borosilicate and lead glasses. Several authors have proposed classification schemes incorporating a number of different analytical techniques for glass examination including SEM/EDX (Reeve *et al.* 1976; Ryland 1986), XRF (Ryland 1986), AA (Hughes *et al.* 1976; Tennent *et al.* 1984), ICP-AES (Hickman 1981, 1987; Becker, Chadzelek and Stoecklein 1999; Almirall *et al.* 1998) and ICP-MS (Wolnik *et al.* 1989; Parouchais *et al.* 1996; Coleman and Goode 1973; Almirall in press; Curran *et al.* 1997a, b).

Although the classification of glass fragments can help as an investigative tool, it is more useful to be able to discriminate between glass samples of the

Table 7.1

Typical values for the elemental concentrations in some glasses (as % of element by weight)

	Si	Na	Ca	Mg	K	Al	Fe	Ba	Pb	B
Silica	99.50 (as SiO2)									
Soda-lime (float)										
(UK)1	34.08	9.50	5.86	2.29	0.66	0.74	0.07			
(US)2	33.90	10.24	6.41	2.29	0.11	0.18	0.12	0.01		
(Germany)2	33.58	10.14	6.60	2.40	0.13	0.28	0.16	0.12		
(Spain)2	33.46	10.24	6.62	2.37	0.21	0.37	0.07			
(Japan)2	33.54	9.66	5.80	2.36	0.83	0.90	0.14			
Soda-lime (container)										
(UK)1	33.99	8.16	9.79	0.06	0.42	0.85	0.03			
Flint (US)1	33.90	10.21	7.10	0.64	0.43	1.04	0.04	0.03		
Green (US)1	33.75	10.29	7.40	0.39	0.46	1.01	0.11	0.04		
Amber(US)1	33.49	10.38	7.25	0.45	0.59	1.31	0.15	0.04		
Borosilicate1	37.55	3.34	0.07		0.25	1.11	0.05			3.82
Lead crystal1	27.39	0.96			10.88		0.01		23.39	0.47

Note: These concentrations reflect the average values for a selected number of plants during the period of 1967–1987. The variation between all glass plants and manufacturers has not been well characterized in the literature due to proprietary concerns.
Sources: (1) Warman, G.P. and Keeley, R.H. *An Introduction to Glass Technology,* MPFSL Report No. 30 and (2) Bell, R.R., *A Use of Commercially Quoted Glass Compositions in Forensic Analysis,* Tech. Note FSL Chefstow, Y89, N0709, September, pp. 1–10.

same type. The ideal analytical technique would distinguish all glass sources. Limitations in analytical methods prevent such individualization of glass fragments. In addition, the manufacturing process of glass objects produces a number of objects having indistinguishable elemental profiles for a given time frame when measured by the current analytical methods. The continuous nature of manufacturing can produce indistinguishable objects within some time frame of the manufacturing process due to the homogeneity of the glass melt. The amount of the homogeneity varies with the type of object, plant, manufacturing cycle and other variables. Fortunately for forensic scientists, there are a great many sources of glass and the methods used to distinguish fragments are sensitive enough to be able to distinguish plant of origin, for example, as well as objects from the same plant at different time intervals.

Absent an alternative explanation for the evidence (such as "the headlamp glass was deposited by another vehicle sporting an identical brand headlamp manufactured in the same manufacturing plant on approximately the same date"), matching profiles for glass samples that did not originate from the same source would be highly unlikely. This statement is supported by two factors: (1) current analytical methods for elemental analysis generate elemental profiles with excellent sensitivity and (2) there is enough variation in the population of possible sources to consider coincidental matches (absent the caveat above) an unusual event. One of the challenges to the forensic scientist is to accurately express this level of "belief" about the evidence and to provide the supporting data for that opinion.

Coleman and Goode (1973) first documented the discrimination potential of elemental composition analysis in glass in 1973 and many publications since then have shown the utility of elemental profiles for discrimination between glass fragments from different sources. A thorough review of the literature on the application of elemental composition analysis to glass examinations can be found in a recent publication (Almirall *et al.* 1998).

Koons *et al.* (1988, 1991) studied the capacity of elemental analysis by ICP-AES to improve the discrimination of glass samples from vehicle windows over RI measurements. These workers examined 81 samples of tempered glass collected from wrecking yards in the Washington DC area. These samples represented 19 makes and 60 models from the period 1974–1987 and there were eight instances of two samples from the same make, model and year of automobile. The authors compared analytical data for the concentrations of Al, Ba, Ca, Fe, Mg, Mn, Na, Sr and Ti. For 81 samples, 3240 possible comparisons are possible, if all samples are to be compared to every other in a pairwise comparison. The authors report that when an RI match criteria of $n_D \pm 0.00020$ is used, 648 of the possible 3240 possible pairs or 20 per cent of the pairs are not distinguishable. They also report that ICP-AES comparisons alone can distinguish all

Table 7.2

Frequency of indistinguishable pairs from 81 different glass samples (3240 possible comparisons).

Comparison parameter and criteria	No. of indistinguishable pairs	Frequency
(1) n_D ±0.0002	648	1:5.0
(2) n_D ±0.0001	418	1:7.8
(3) (1) and n_C ±0.0004 and n_F ±0.0004	487	1:6.7
(4) (2) and n_C ±0.0002 and n_F ±0.0002	178	1:18.2
(5) EDXRF	305	1:10.6
(6) (5) and (3)	81	1:40
(7) (5) and (4)	33	1:98
(8) ICP-AES	3	1:1080
(9) (8) and (3)	3	1:1080
(10) (8) and (4)	2	1:1620

Source: Koons *et al.* (1991) *Journal of Analytical Atomic Spectroscopy*, 6, 451–456.

but three of the 3240 pairs (0.09 per cent of the pairs are not distinguished). Table 7.2 summarizes the results from the comparisons based on different match criteria used for the comparison. The three samples that were indistinguishable originated from the same make (Ford Motor Company), and the models Thunderbird, Lincoln Mark IV and Lincoln Mark V, all produced in the model year 1977. Since Ford manufactured all the vehicles in the same year, the results suggest a single source of production for the glass.

ELEMENTAL ANALYSIS OF HEADLAMP GLASS

The elemental composition of headlamp glass is very different from the composition of the soda-lime glasses. The metals Al, Fe and Zr are present in concentrations well above the detection limits of the method and these elements provide good discrimination potential. A pairwise comparison of the same 60 headlamps that were evaluated by RI were also evaluated (Almirall *et al.* 1996) by the analysis of Al, Fe, Zr, Mg, Ca, and Ti concentrations. Index comparisons did not distinguish 654 of the 1770 possible pairs. When the above elements were analyzed by ICP-AES and compared, 12 of the 1770 pairs (0.68 per cent of the possible pairs) were not distinguished.

METHODOLOGY

The analytical method used for the quantitative analysis of the glass samples in this case was atomic emission spectroscopy with inductively coupled argon plasma as an excitation source (ICP-AES). This method was chosen over other quantitative techniques due to its sensitivity, precision and accuracy for the range of concentrations of the elements of interest. The procedure in this case was modified from a method previously described by Koons *et al.* (1988).

STATISTICAL ANALYSIS OF GLASS DATA

Unlike other materials of transfer evidence, glass measurements and comparisons provide continuous (quantitative) data that can be used in comparison schemes. Paint and fiber comparisons consist of class characteristics that may be reduced to discrete categorical data such as color, polymer type (even though RI is sometimes used in classifying fibers), number of layers, etc. Refractive index and elemental composition data are a result of measurements taken with analytical techniques with known precision and accuracy limitations. Conventional descriptive statistical tools are used to examine those limitations and the potential error associated with the measurements. Descriptive statistics are also used to describe the population and to present the data in an easily understandable manner. Methods in hypothesis testing are used as a means to draw inferences from the data.

CASE RESULTS

Three glass fragments that were removed from the vehicle were analyzed by ICP-AES. Quantitative analysis of the metals Al, Fe, Zr, Mg, Ca, and Ti were performed. The three fragments had mean concentrations of 1011.9 µg g^{-1} for Al, 18.2 µg g^{-1} for Fe, 98.6 µg g^{-1} for Zr, 7.1 µg g^{-1} for Mg, 88.4 µg g^{-1} for Ca and 15.8 µg g^{-1} for Ti. The standard deviations were determined to be 13.7 µg g^{-1}, 1.0 µg g^{-1}, 4.8 µg g^{-1}, 0.4 µg g^{-1}, 8.2 µg g^{-1} and 2.1 µg g^{-1} for Al, Fe, Zr, Mg, Ca, and Ti respectively.

Three fragments recovered from the scene of the accident were also analyzed by ICP-AES and using a range overlap comparison criteria where ± 2 SD from the mean of the standards constituted the range, the fragments recovered from the scene could not be distinguished from the standard fragments.

CASE CONCLUSIONS

In an attempt to determine the actual number of possible contributors of the glass on the island, I requested a list of registered vehicles from the police department but they were not able to provide it.

A report was written based on the visual observations, the RI and elemental analysis results. The report summarized the results by stating that based on the comparison between the standard fragments and the fragments recovered from the scene "[these results] indicate that these fragments originated from the same headlamp or a similar headlamp". A preliminary hearing was held to present the evidence and during the testimony, I was able to summarize that the results of the glass analysis were strong evidence for the association between the glass fragments. Days before the full trial was to take place, the crown prosecutor and defense reached an agreement but the terms of the agreement were not provided.

FUTURE WORK IN GLASS ANALYSIS
INDUCTIVELY COUPLED PLASMA–MASS SPECTROMETRY

Since this case was completed, a standard method for the elemental analysis of glass by ICP-MS has been developed and tested through a series of round-robin studies. The research that led to the development and publication of the method (Duckworth *et al.* 2000) was funded by the National Institute of Justice for a collaborative study between the Oak Ridge National Laboratory and the International Forensic Research Institute at Florida International University. ICP-MS combines the multi-element capability and the broad dynamic range of ICP emission with the enhanced sensitivity and ability to perform quantitative analyses of the elemental isotopic concentrations and ratios. The enhanced sensitivity allows for the analysis of smaller fragments (as low as 500 µg) and the isotopic analysis capability permits isotope dilution experiments that would improve the precision of the method further.

Suzuki *et al.* (1997) recently reported the discrimination of 22 windshield glass samples by pairwise comparison of the elements Co, Rb, Sr, Zr, Ba, La and Ce. All 231 pairs could be discriminated by composition and RI comparisons while 15 pairs were indistinguishable by RI comparison only. These workers also report the successful discrimination of all 138 pairs of 17 samples of headlamp glasses by comparison of the Zr, Ba, Sr, Sb, Hf, As, Mo and Pb concentrations and RI while 19 pairs could not be discriminated by RI comparison alone. Suzuki *et al.* (2000) also reported the complete discrimination of all 120 possible pairs of 16 container glass samples (bottles) by ICP-MS using elemental composition (Co, Cu, Zn, Rb, Sr, Zr, Ag, Sn, Sb, Ba, La, Ce and Pb) when 13 of the pairs were indistinguishable using RI only.

Recent studies by Stoecklein *et al.* (1996, 1998) and Becker *et al.* (1999) of 61 glass samples from 45 float plants representing the US, Europe and Asia glass productions produced 1830 possible pairwise comparisons. These workers report 100 per cent discrimination by measuring the composition of 30 elements and a range overlap criteria (comparing the mean ± 2 SD). These workers report the most useful elements for discrimination to be Al, K, Ti, Mn, Fe, Rb, Sr, Zr, Sn, Bi, Sb, Eu, Ho and Pb.

The author is currently developing a large database of elemental profiles including a variety of glass types (float glass from windows of different types, containers, headlamps, cookware, and leaded glass) by multi-element ICP-MS and Isotope Dilution (ID)-ICP-MS. It is expected that this data will further demonstrate the utility of elemental composition analysis for glass discrimination.

ACKNOWLEDGEMENTS

I would like to thank the late Dr Bill Hartner of the MDPD crime laboratory for assistance and guidance during my tenure at the MDPD crime laboratory. I also want to thank Professor Michael Cole of the Forensic Science Unit of the University of Strathclyde for his technical guidance during aspects in my research on glass and Professor Rosemary Hickey-Vargas of the Department of Geology of FIU for allowing the MDPD to use the ICP-AES located in her laboratory. Finally, I want to thank the National Institute of Justice for financial support to research in glass examinations.

REFERENCES

Almirall, J.R. (in press) "Elemental analysis of glass fragments", in *Trace Evidence Analysis and Interpretation: Glass and Paint*, ed. B Caddy, Taylor and Francis.

Almirall, J., Cole, M., Furton, K., and Gettinby, G. (1996) "Characterization of glass evidence by the statistical analysis of their inductively coupled plasma/atomic emission spectroscopy and refractive index data," *Proceedings of the American Academy of Forensic Sciences Meeting, Nashville, TN,* 19–24 February, 2, p. 50.

Almirall, J.R., Cole, M., Furton, K.G., and Gettinby, G. (1998) "Discrimination of glass sources using elemental composition and refractive index: development of predictive models," *Science and Justice*, 38 (2), 93–100.

Almirall, J.R., Buckleton, J., Curran, J., and Hicks, T. (2000) "Examination of glass" in *Forensic Interpretation of Glass Evidence*, ed. J. Curran, T. Hicks, and J. Buckleton, CRC Press, pp. 1–26.

Association of Official Analytical Chemists (1990) "Characterization and matching of glass fragments", *Official Methods of Analysis,* vol. 973.65, pp. 637–639.

ASTM (2000) *ASTM 1967–98, Standard Test Method for the Automated Determination of Refractive Index of Glass Samples Using the Oil Immersion Method and a Phase Contrast*

Microscope, in 2000 Annual Book of ASTM Standards, vol. 14.02, American Society for Testing and Materials, Philadelphia, PA, pp. 819–821.

Becke, F. (1892) "Tschermak's Mineralogische und Petrographische Mitteilungen," *MPMTA,* 13, 379–430.

Becker, S., Chadzelek, A., and Stoecklein, W. (1999) "Classification of float glasses with respect to their origin by chemometric analysis of elemental concentrations and the use of LA-ICP-MS as a tool in forensic science," *Proceedings of European Winter Conference on Plasma Spectrochemistry*, Pau, France, pp. 113–114.

Cassista, A.R. and Sandercock, P.M.L. (1994) "Precision of glass refractive index measurements: temperature variation and double variation methods, and the value of dispersion," *Canadian Society of Forensic Science*, 27, 203–208.

Coleman, R., and Goode, G. (1973) "Comparison of glass fragments by neutron activation analysis," *Journal of Radioanalytical Chemistry*, 15, 367–388.

Collins, B. and Kobus, H.K. (1987) "Automatic glass refractive index muasurement using GRIM; an evaluation of the system," personal communication.

Curran, J., Triggs, C., Almirall, J.R., Buckleton, J., and Walsh, K. (1997a) "The interpretation of elemental composition measurements from forensic glass," *Science and Justice; Journal of the Forensic Science Society*, 37(4), 241–245.

Curran, J., Triggs, C., Almirall, J.R., Buckleton, J., and Walsh, K. (1997b) "The interpretation of elemental composition measurements from forensic glass II," *Science and Justice; Journal of the Forensic Science Society*, 37(4), 245–249.

Duckworth, D.C., Bayne, C.K., Morton, S.J., and Almirall, J.R. (2000) "Analysis of variance in forensic glass analysis by ICP-MS: variance within the method," *Journal of Analytical and Atomic Spectrometry,* 15(7), 821–828.

Hickman, D. A. (1981) "A classification scheme for glass," *Forensic Science International,* 17, 265–281.

Hickman, D. A. (1987) "Glass types identified by chemical analysis," *Forensic Science International*, 33, 23–46.

Hughes, J., Catterick, T., and Southeard, G. (1976) "The quantitative analysis of glass by atomic absorption spectroscopy," *Journal of Forensic Sciences*, 8, 217-227.

Johnson, R.A. and Wichern, D.W. (1992) *Applied Multivariate Statistical Analysis*, 3rd edition, Prentice Hall, Inc., pp. 522–533.

Koons, R.D., Fiedler, C., and Rawalt, R. (1988) "Classification and discrimination of sheet and container glasses by inductively coupled plasma-atomic emission spectrometry and pattern recognition," *Journal of Forensic Sciences,* 33(1), 49–67.

Koons, R., Peters, C., and Rebbert, P. (1991) "Comparison of refractive index, energy dispersive x-ray fluorescence and inductively coupled plasma atomic emission spectrometry for
forensic characterization of sheet glass fragments," *Journal of Analytical Atomic Spectrometry*, 6, 451–456.

Locke, J. (1985) "The determination of glass refractive index using GRIM – a collaborative
exercise," personal communication.

Ojena, S.M. and De Forest, P.R. (1972) "A study of the refractive index variations within and
between sealed beam headlamps using a precise method," *Journal of Forensic Sciences*,
12, 315–329.

Parouchais, T., Warner, I., Palmer, L., and Kobus, H. (1996) "The analysis of small glass
fragments using inductively coupled plasma mass spectrometry," *Journal of Forensic
Sciences*, 41, 351–360.

Reeve, V., Mathieson, J., and Fong, W. (1976) "Elemental analysis by energy dispersive X-ray:
a significant factor in the forensic analysis of glass," *Journal of Forensic Sciences*, 21,
291–306.

Ryland, S.G. (1986) "Sheet or container? Forensic glass comparisons with an emphasis on
source classification," *Journal of Forensic Sciences*, 31 (4), 1314–1329.

Stocklein, W., Kubassek, E., Fischer, R., and Chadzelek, A. (1996) "The forensic analysis of
float-glass characterization of glasses from international sources," Forensic Science
Institute, BKA, *Trace Evidence Meeting*, San Antonio, July.

Stoecklein, W., Fischer, R., Becker, S., and Chadzelek, A. (1997) *International Workshop on the
Forensic Examination of Trace Evidence*, Tokyo, pp. 71–79.

Suzuki, Y., Sugita, R., Suzuki, S., and Kishi, T. (1997) "Application of ICP-MS for the forensic
discrimination of glass fragments," *Proceedings of The American Academy of Forensic
Sciences Meeting*, New York, NY, 17–22 February, vol. 3, p. 43.

Suzuki, Y., Sugita, R., Suzuki, S., and Marumo, Y. (2000) "Forensic discrimination of bottle
glass by refractive index measurement and analysis of trace elements with ICP-MS," *Analytical Science*, 16(11), 1195–1198.

Tennent, N., McKenna, P., Lo, K., and Ottaway, J. (1984) "Major, minor and trace element
analysis of medieval stained glass by flame atomic absorption spectrometry," in *Archaeological Chemistry*, ed. J. Lambert, ACS Advances in Chemistry Series no. 205, American
Chemical Society, pp. 133–150.

Wolnik, K., Gaston, C., and Fricke, F. (1989) "Analysis of glass in product tampering investigations by inductively coupled plasma atomic emission spectrometry with a hydrofluoric
acid resistant torch," *Journal of Analytical Atomic Spectrometry*, 4, 27–31.

CHAPTER 8

FEATHERS

Lee Brun-Conti

INTRODUCTION

Trace evidence can come in the form of any number of things. In 13 years as a trace evidence analyst, the author has encountered ball-bearing grease (used in a sexual assault), a golf club head, cat food, spaghetti sauce, cooked meat, and animal feces as trace evidence. Even though most of the items submitted as evidence are items that are mass-produced, the associative value of trace evidence is irrefutable. With the advent and popularity of DNA, the courts, investigators, and some labs are becoming shortsighted, thinking that DNA will make the case and any other evidence is redundant. Make no mistake, DNA is a very powerful biological tool and the advances in DNA technology are amazing; however, it cannot stand alone. A positive DNA match holds no weight if it can be explained away, if "reasonable doubt" exists such as consensual sex or resuscitating a dying person.

THE CRIME SCENE AND THE INVESTIGATION

In the late fall of 1990, two men were driving to work at approximately 6.00 a.m. when they noticed something along the north side of the road. At first they thought that it was a dummy that someone had thrown in the brush, possibly stolen from a house as a Halloween prank. They got out of their car for a closer inspection and discovered that it was a person, an African-American male lying face down in the leaves, wearing tan pants and a blue down jacket. The victim had died violently. They notified the police. Upon arriving at the scene, the detectives from the local police department decided that it would be in the best interest of the investigation to contact the State Police crime laboratory for assistance.

The body was found in a large bedroom community northwest of a major Michigan city. It is a somewhat up-scale, quiet community that is not used to violent crimes. The crime laboratory personnel that arrived at the scene consisted of a latent print examiner, a firearms examiner, and a trace evidence examiner. The road was a half-mile north of the area's major shopping mall;

despite all the traffic to and from the mall, this quiet dirt road was barely notice-able (Figures 8.1a–8.1d). The items of evidence were inventoried and plotted on a grid. The scene was photographed, then bright yellow plastic tents with numbers on them were used to mark where items of evidence were found. The scene was then re-photographed to better show the relationship of the evidence to the victim. A number of items, such as a lighter, a pack of cigarettes, cigarette butts, and empty beer bottles, which may have seemed insignificant as miscella-neous items that would be found as garbage along any road, were collected; at a crime scene nothing should be ignored. More obvious items that were almost certainly connected to the crime, such as suspected blood droplets in the dirt on the road, a wristwatch, and a gray knit cap were also collected. All these items were collected prior to the examination of the victim's body.

The victim was lying on his stomach. A large amount of blood was visible on his upper thigh, near his buttocks, that had soaked through his pants. His down jacket had been cut in many places, which scattered the down along the side of the road; but no blood-soaked areas could be seen. When the victim was turned over, a large stain of blood on the inside front of the down jacket, a small spot of

Figure 8.1
The crime scene.

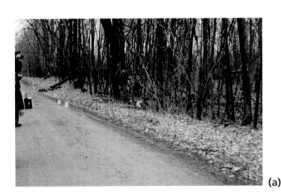
(a)

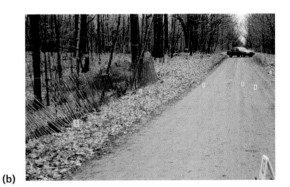
(b)

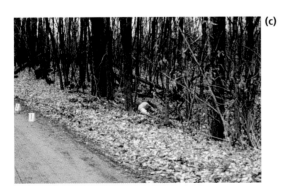
(c)

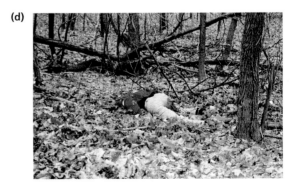
(d)

blood near his crotch, and small bloodstains on his pants could be seen. When the representative of the medical examiner's office arrived, the victim was taken to the county morgue for an autopsy.

The results of the autopsy showed that the victim had met his end in a violent fashion. He was stabbed over eleven times. His wounds included gashes to his left arm, stab wounds to his right side, upper left chest, between his shoulder blades and through-and-through stab wounds to the rear of his right thigh through to his scrotum, and through his right arm. There was also a gash on his right hand that ran the length of his hand. Defense wounds could be seen on his hands showing that the victim did not die without a struggle. The cause of death was from multiple stab wounds. What happened to bring this man to such a savage end? The local police were already beginning to piece the events leading to the crime together.

The victim's name was Dennis Kennedy,[1] but he was more commonly known as Rick. He lived with his father in a suburb of Detroit about 10 miles east of the crime scene. Detectives visited the home of the victim's father to question him about the events that occurred the last time that he had seen his son alive. According to the father, he had driven his son to his son's girlfriend's house in Detroit the evening before the body was found because Rick's car was broken down at the time.

The detectives paid a visit to Rick's girlfriend; she said that Rick had received a phone call from a man with a Hispanic accent and that Rick had left. Through their investigation the detectives learned that Rick's sister was once married to a Cuban named Donato Montoya so they decided to question him next. Upon arriving at the home of Montoya they found no one home and left a note for him to contact the local Police Department. Montoya later contacted the police and arranged for an interview.

During the first interview Montoya told the police almost all of the truth regarding the events of the night of the crime. But during the first interview with Montoya, two potential suspects were mentioned: Cubans named Nicholas Cortez and Franco Portas who had come to the Detroit area from the west side of the state in search of drugs. The detectives then contacted police agencies on the west side of the state for assistance in locating Cortez and Portas. The detectives also obtained information on the type of vehicle that Cortez and Portas were driving and the vehicle in which Montoya last saw Rick alive: a gray Lincoln Continental.

Meanwhile, the Michigan State Police crime lab personnel were processing the evidence recovered from the crime scene and the autopsy. The bloodstains recovered from the road were type O and hairs found in the gray cap were consistent with the victim; therefore neither could be eliminated as having a different source than the victim. The cigarette butt did not show any serological

[1] All names have been changed.

evidence of coming from any specific blood type; the victim, however, was not a secretor. Eighty per cent of the population has secretor status: their blood type is revealed through other body fluids, such as saliva or semen. Even if the victim did smoke the cigarette, no blood group substances would have been found on it. The cigarette butt, pack of cigarettes, and beer bottles were processed for latent prints. Some latent prints were found on these items but were not the victim's and were not of sufficient quality to be entered into the Automated Fingerprint Identification System (AFIS). The watch recovered was later discovered to belong to the victim, a gift from his brother, but was not working at the time. This was, apparently, the reason that the victim was wearing a second wristwatch when he was killed. The items submitted for trace evidence analysis were the victim's clothing, a book of matches, the watch the victim was wearing, the victim's clothing, and an "Oldsmobile" hood ornament. Nothing submitted to the trace evidence section was perceived to have any apparent evidential value. This perception would later prove false.

The police investigation continued. Nicholas Cortez was apprehended at his girlfriend's house on the west side of the state and his vehicle was impounded. Cortez's car, a 1983 Cadillac Eldorado, was parked in a tow-away zone outside of his girlfriend's apartment. Per departmental policy, an impounded vehicle must be searched and an inventory taken; the reason for this is for civil liability. If the car was impounded and the owner said that there were $4000 in it and the money was not there upon the car's return, a lawsuit could ensue. The police found an interesting item in the trunk: a pair of bloodstained pants. These pants, along with Nicholas Cortez, were turned over to the local police.

The pants were brought to the crime lab where they were examined. Bloodstains from two different sources were found on the pants. One stain was consistent with blood type A and the other, smaller stain was consistent with type O. Known blood from all the individuals involved was submitted for typing; as it turned out, the victim, Cortez, Portas, and Montoya all had type O blood. The known blood from the victim and a swatch of the bloodstained pants were sent to a private laboratory for DNA testing. The results of the analysis showed that the type O blood on the jeans was from the victim. However, this biological evidence was far removed from the crime scene. Even though it was found in the car of one of the suspects, it was not the vehicle that Montoya remembered last seeing the victim, Cortez and Portas in. What if the suspects said that they had just gotten into a little scuffle with Rick and had then dropped him off somewhere? What if the suspects contended that Rick attacked them and they, while fending him off, got some of his blood on their jeans? The detectives thought that they needed more physical evidence putting Cortez and/or Portas at the scene. They needed to find the Lincoln Continental.

The police interviewed Montoya again. Montoya told the same story as was given in the first interview. In the third interview, however, Montoya finally told the truth. His story ran as follows.

Prior to the death of the victim, Cortez contacted Montoya by phone wanting to know where he could buy a kilo of cocaine. Montoya contacted the victim. As stated before, Montoya was once married to the victim's sister and even though the marriage ended, the friendship between the men didn't. They would get together a few times a week to work on cars. Montoya knew that the victim both used and sold drugs and that the victim had asked Montoya on a number of occasions if he knew anyone who wanted to buy drugs. So when Cortez called and said that he needed to be hooked up with a kilo of cocaine and that he, Cortez, had $27,000 to spend, Montoya knew whom to contact. Besides, Montoya thought that his trouble might be worth about a grand.

Cortez said that he would be coming into town with his friend Franco. Montoya also knew Franco through Franco's brother but did not know Franco's last name. Cortez and Franco drove over to the Detroit area from the west side of the state. They got a room at a local hotel, had a bite to eat in the restaurant, and arranged to meet Montoya. Since neither Cortez nor Franco knew the area very well, Montoya decided to drive them in their vehicle, a gray Lincoln Continental. The three men, Montoya driving, Franco in the front passenger's seat, and Cortez in the passenger's side rear seat, went to meet up with the victim by a restaurant. After waiting 15 or 20 minutes, the victim Rick showed up and got in the back seat with Cortez, sitting behind Montoya. The four men drove, being directed by the victim, from one drug house to another. After finding no success at four consecutive stops, the victim decided to discuss the value of the cocaine that he was trying to obtain for Cortez and Franco. The victim said that a kilo was worth $28,000 and they only had $27,000. After the discussion regarding the price of a kilo, apparently Cortez and Franco thought that the victim (Rick) could do nothing for them so they brought him back to his girlfriend's house.

Montoya, Cortez, and Portas discussed what they would do next. Rick couldn't get them their drugs at the price that they wanted to pay but what could they do? They didn't know anyone else who could obtain drugs for them. They decided to call Rick back and have him try a few more of his sources. Rick made some more calls and finally contacted someone who would sell a kilo of cocaine for $27,000. The dealer said that he would meet the men at a local hamburger place.

After waiting for about an hour the dealer finally arrived and the transaction was about to begin. The dealer told Rick to meet him behind the Mobile gas station where they had a discussion for about ten minutes. Rick returned and said that they would just exchange "packages" and then both parties would leave. Portas opened the trunk of his car and Cortez removed the small canvas bag containing the $27,000. All four men walked over to the dealer's car and conducted the transaction through the passenger's side door. A package of what was thought to be a kilo of cocaine was sitting on the passenger's seat. The package was wrapped very tightly with a lot of tape. Cortez tried to see into the package with no luck. Montoya was getting nervous so to move things along he took the bag with the money from Cortez and gave it to the dealer. The dealer took off with the money, leaving the four men with their package. They walked back to the Lincoln and Cortez, now in the front seat, dug at the package trying to open it. Finally, using his key, Cortez opened the package and saw that it was sugar. He said, in Spanish, "This is not what it's supposed to be."

Cortez said that no one was leaving the car until he got the cocaine or his money back. Rick suggested that the group attempt to find the person that ripped them off and get their money back. All agreed and as they were about to begin their search, Cortez asked Montoya if he had any weapons. Montoya said that the only weapon that he had was a knife, which was at his apartment. The group drove to Montoya's apartment and got the knife. Montoya returned to the car with the knife in his waistband.

The four men drove around the west side of the city, going to at least three different houses, looking for the dealer and their money. By 10.30 p.m. they were no closer to getting their money back. Rick said that he needed to eat immediately but Cortez reiterated that no one was leaving the car until the money or the cocaine was found. Cortez and Franco, who were more fluent in Spanish than English, began speaking to each other increasingly in Spanish. Although Montoya could understand them, Rick could not. Cortez and Franco had begun to suspect that Rick had set them up. "Tenemos que ponerle precion" ("We have to put pressure on him"), said Cortez. "Si, berdad tu tienes razon" ("Yes, that is the truth"), responded Franco. Cortez and Franco were beginning to get more and more suspicious of Rick.

Cortez then said, "Tu tienes domarlo" ("We have to tame him"). This is not a phrase that is normally used in reference to humans; it is usually used to describe what is done to animals. Montoya described feeling that Cortez was going to harm Rick when he made the last statement. Rick again insisted that he needed something to eat. Rick and Cortez argued.

At this point Montoya insisted on being dropped off at home, because he said that his wife would be worried about him. In truth, Montoya had sent his wife and one-year-old son to stay at his aunt's house because, he told her, he was going to be involved in something and he didn't want to endanger either her or the child. Montoya felt that things were going to get a lot worse between Cortez, Franco, and Rick and he wanted no part of that. Montoya drove the car to his apartment. At some point during the evening Montoya removed his knife from his waistband and set it on the floorboard of the Lincoln. As Montoya was leaving the vehicle, Cortez and Franco asked for directions to get back home. The directions that Montoya gave them sent them about one and a half miles from where the body of the victim would be found the next morning.

Montoya got into his apartment and immediately called his wife to come pick him up. He instructed her not to come to the apartment but to pick him up a few blocks down the street. When she saw Montoya he was visibly upset and he related the evening's events to her.

Exactly what happened to the victim after Montoya left him, Cortez, and Franco will probably never be known. But what is known is that Dennis "Rick" Kennedy died on that dirt road during the night of November 8 or the early morning hours of November 9.

The morning of November 9, Nicholas Cortez contacted Montoya and wanted him to put up signs on the houses that they had gone to on the previous night trying to locate the cocaine or their money. The signs would read "Return the money, or else". Montoya told Cortez that he would do that but in actual fact he never did put the signs up. Cortez called Montoya a second time asking "Si, lo entrotraro roto?" ("If they had found him broken [yet]?"). Cortez told Montoya not to say anything to anybody and to remember that the knife that they had in the car belonged to Montoya. This last statement by Cortez explained why it took the detectives three interviews to get the whole story from Montoya. Remembering the threat and that the knife, which obviously was used to kill Rick, belonged to him, Montoya was afraid to give the whole story to the police. But he did give the police enough information for a warrant for Cortez and Franco.

The police discovered the last name of Franco through Cortez's brother: Portas. Now that the police knew his full name, they could now arrest him and confiscate his car, the Lincoln Continental that Montoya remembered from the night of November 8.

When the Lincoln was impounded the police brought it to the Michigan State Police Crime Laboratory. Upon initial examination of the vehicle, it was noticed that the back of the front passenger seat was missing. The seat itself was similar to a bucket seat and the piece that was missing was the rear of the seat. Using book tape, the front and rear seats, which were leather, were taped to collect any trace evidence. Known carpet fiber samples from the floor carpeting and floor mats were also collected. The inside of the car was processed for latent prints. The hood of the car was opened and a piece of bird down was found stuck in the center of the radiator. This piece of down was collected as evidence.

One latent print was found in the car located on a plastic card that was tucked into the trim above the windshield. The print was identified as having come from Nicholas Cortez. Therefore, Nicholas Cortez was either once in the vehicle or at one time touched the card that was found in the vehicle. The victim's clothing from the autopsy was submitted and the known fibers from the victim's outer clothing, the tan pants, and the blue down jacket were compared with any questioned fibers recovered from the fibers on the tape lifts from the Lincoln. No fibers were found on the tape lifts that were consistent with the victim's outer clothing. The victim's shoes were also examined for carpet fibers consistent with the carpet or floor mats from the Lincoln; none were found. The last item to be examined was the piece of down recovered from the radiator of the Lincoln.

ANALYSIS

The initial examination of the down began with a microscopic comparison with the down from the victim's jacket. The feathers appeared similar and were consistent with the down from a duck or goose (Chandler 1916; Robertson *et al.* 1982). Knowledge of the types, anatomy, and function of bird feathers is crucial to a proper identification and comparison of feathers. It is also important to understand how feathers are processed for use in clothing and textiles.

A representative from United Feather and Down was contacted for information about the use of down in clothing. United Feather and Down get most of their down from Europe. The down is washed with soap and water repeatedly, dried (but not exposed to a lot of heat), cooled, and then bagged. Four grades of down are machine-sorted: down, half down (which is 15 per cent down), C-feathers (feathers under four inches long), and large feathers (feathers over four inches long which are crushed). Occasionally some manufacturers use chicken or turkey feathers or down to supplement less expensive products.

There are six commonly recognized types of bird feathers: contour feathers, down, semiplume, filoplume, bristle, and powder down (Figure 8.2). No matter the type of feather, unless it is growing on a young bird or after a molt, the feather does not have any living cells; it is a dead, horny structure made of keratin. The feather that we commonly think of when we think of feathers is a contour feather. Contour feathers not only cover the bird's body but are also the flight feathers. Flight feathers (on the wing) can be distinguished from the contour feathers covering the body by the fact that the vanes on flight feathers are asymmetrical and the leading edge of the feather has short, tightly bound barbs tough enough to head into the wind, whereas the trailing barbs are longer and will bend upward to provide lift and forward movement (Figure 8.3).

Starting proximally the first part of the contour feather is the inferior umbilicus, which is attached to the bird. This structure provides nourishment to the growing feather and is used to attach the feather securely to the bird once the feather is full-grown. The next portion up is the calamus or quill. Further up is the superior umbilicus, which is the juncture where the calamus becomes the

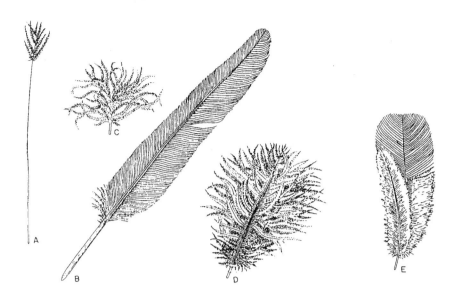

Figure 8.2

Types of feathers. A, filolume; B, vane or contour; C, down; D, semiplume; E, contour feather with aftershaft (bristles and powder down not shown). (From J. C. Welty, The Life of Birds)

rachis, and the two webs of vane form. Also at the point of the superior umbilicus is a structure that is common to many birds, called an aftershaft. The aftershaft is usually small and downy in most birds, however, there are the exceptions, like in the emu which has an aftershaft as long as the main feather. The webs of the vane, along with the rachis, form a light, flexible, and flat structure that is necessary for flight. The rachis is grooved on its inner surface (the surface close to the bird's body) and is flat on its side so that the cross-section of the rachis looks like a square. The web of the vane is made up of barbs called rami. There

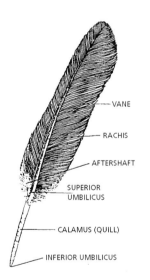

Figure 8.3

The parts of a typical contour feather. (From J. C. Welty, The Life of Birds)

can be hundreds of rami on each web and they are attached to the flat edge of the rachis. Rami will be stiffer near the tip of the wing and softer near the base. The microscopic structure of the rami is quite interesting. The reason you can split the rami or barbs of the web of the vane but if you run your finger up from the bottom to the top along that web then the web returns to a seamless unit is that the barb or rami has microscopic structures called barbules or radii on

Figure 8.4

*Hooklets and smooth
barbules from a contour
feather of a partridge.*

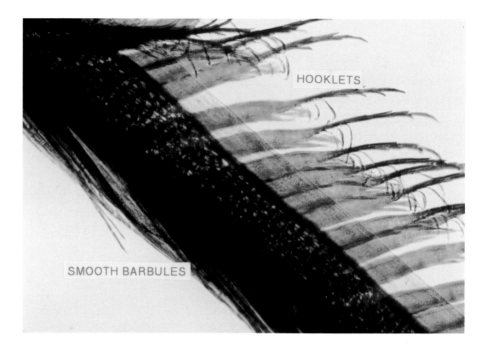

each side of the barb. On the distal side of the barb (the side near the tip of the feather) are hooklets. As the name implies, hooklets look like tiny hooks. On the proximal side of the barb (the side near the base of the feather) there are smooth barbules that are like rods. The distal hooklet from one barb will hook onto the smooth barbule from the next barb resulting in a seamless or unbroken web. This part of the feather is called the pennaceous region (Figure 8.4).

The last feature on the contour feather is the small tufts of down near the base of the vane. This will be discussed later, as the examination of these downy barbules is important to discovering the taxonomy of the feather.

Down feathers are fluffy because they have no hooklets to hook onto smooth barbules; therefore, they form no seamless web. The down feather has only a slender rachia. They are similar to the downy barbules at the base of the contour feather. Down is usually concealed under the contour feathers in adult birds (except in Old World Vultures in which the exposed down around the neck makes them look like they are wearing a fur collar). The young of some birds are covered in down but the structure and texture of this down differs from adult down which is primarily used for warmth. Therefore it doesn't come as a surprise that down is in great abundance in water birds such as gulls, ducks, geese, penguins, and pelicans.

Semiplume feathers are the intermediaries between contour feathers and down. These feathers have a rachis and barbs but no hooklets or smooth barbules so they remain fluffy. They are found under the contour feathers on the sides of the abdomen, neck and mid-back and they provide insulation as well as flexibility and increased buoyancy. The marabou used to make boas are semiplumes.

Filoplumes are hair-like feathers that usually grow in groups of two to eight at the base of a contour feather. There are two types of filoplumes: one has a small vane at the top and the other has no vane at all. Filoplumes are usually covered by contour feathers, particularly the mechanically active flight feathers. It is suspected that filoplumes are associated with the sensory functions that control feather movement because the follicles surrounding the filoplumes are supplied with an abundance of nerve endings.

Small vaneless contour feathers are known as bristles. These consist of a small, stiff rachis and few if any barbs. The functions of bristles are to protect against dirt and dust, as in the eyelashes of the ostrich, or in a tactile function.

Powder down is a specialized form of down which grows continuously and is never molted. It produces a waxy powder that is used for waterproofing and dressing of the plumage. The tips of the powder down disintegrate into small (about one micron) water-resistant particles that are scattered throughout the plumage while the bird is preening. In some birds, the powder from the powder down will add a metallic-like luster to the feathers.

The most distinctive down, the down that will help the most with the taxonomic identification of the feather, is the down found at the base of the contour feathers. All but the most specialized contour feathers have a downy portion. Down is made up of barbs coming off the rachis and barbules that are both distal and proximal on the barbs. These barbules lack hooks and therefore do not have a pennaceous structure. The down from a waterfowl is very tightly attached to the body of the bird. This information added weight to the argument that the down found in the radiator of the suspect's vehicle was not from a source in the wild. Along the barbules are structures called nodes, which are swollen areas at varying intervals along the barbule. Depending upon the species of the bird, these nodes will take on different shapes. Robertson *et al.* (1982) classify the nodes into six different shapes: expanded, pronged, ring, vase-shaped, triangular, and quadrilobe.

The expanded node is found on most species of birds. The only information that can be gained from expanded nodes is if they are missing, in which case the feather may be from the order *Falconiformes* (eagles, falcons, and hawks with the exception of the kestrel) (Figure 8.5).

Pronged nodes are also quite common in many orders of birds that also have nodes of other shapes present. However, in the order *Falconiformes*, when pronged nodes are present, they are asymmetrical. These are the only nodes present in this order (except for the kestrel that has only a slight swelling, a hint of an expanded node along the length of the barbule) (Figure 8.6).

Figure 8.5
*Expanded node from a
macaw (400×).*

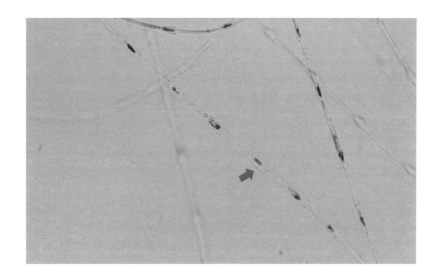

Figure 8.6

A pronged node from a
Falconiforme *(400×).*
*The schematic shows the
configuration of a
pronged node from a* Fal-
coniforme. *(Schematic
drawing from M. G. Day,*
Identification of Hair
and Feather Remains
in the Gut and Faeces
of Stoats and Weasels)

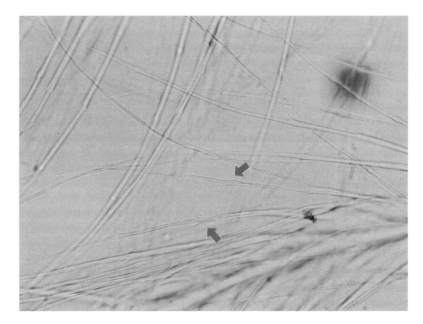

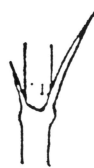

Ring nodes are found in the order *Galliformes* (chickens, pheasants, and turkeys) and, as the name implies, appear to be a ring around the barbule. Ring nodes may look like vase-shaped nodes (described below) with a curled lip on the vase. In these cases it is useful to focus the microscope stage up and down to see the three-dimensional appearance of the ring. The ring node is interesting in that sometimes a ring will "slip off" and slide down the barbule and get caught on the ring adjacent to it (Figure 8.7).

Vase-shaped nodes are found in the order *Passeriformes*, which constitutes about 50 per cent of the bird population (Chandler 1916). *Passeriformes* consist of perching birds like robins, blue jays, and chickadees. The nodes are usually pigmented. Another structure that is present in *Passeriformes* is a finger-like protrusion at the base of the barbule called villi (Figure 8.8).

Triangular nodes are found in the orders *Psittaciformes* (or order *Cuculiformes*, suborders *Cuculi* and *Psittici*, being cuckoos and parrots, respectively) and *Anseriformes*. These two may be distinguished from each other because the triangular nodes on the down from the *Anseriformes* appear to be a smoother triangle along a thin barbule. The nodes from the *Psittaciformes* have sharper points and the barbule is not as thin as that of the *Anseriforme* (Figure 8.9).

Columbiformes (or order *Charadriiformes*, suborder *Pteroclocolumbae* depending upon the reference), consisting of pigeons and doves in the group Columbae, have quadrilobed nodes (Figure 8.10).

Most migrating waterfowl will have left southeastern Michigan or will be going south by November unless they have a source of food and running water (Wood 1951). If the waterfowl have these basic needs then they have no reason to migrate. The common Canada goose (*Branta canadensis canadensis*) migrates

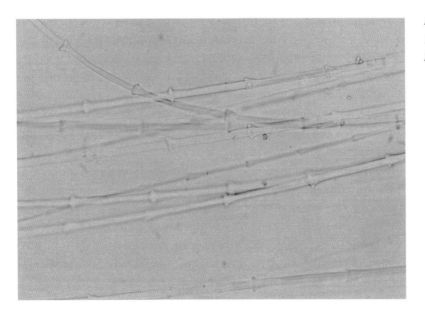

Figure 8.7
Ring node from a partridge (400×).

Figure 8.8
Vase-shaped node from a finch (400×).

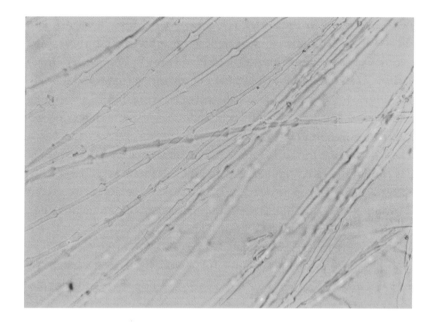

from Michigan's Lower Peninsula from October to mid-November. The common Mallard (*Anas platyrhynchos platyrhynchos*) also migrates south in October and November. The location of the homicide is at the edge of an area known for its lakes and there are hundreds in that area, some of which may not freeze over in the winter. The area near the crime scene is known for having ducks and geese all year.

Ducks and geese will molt all of their primary, or wing feathers, at once as opposed to tree-perching birds that lose their flight feathers in a regular sequential pattern (Welty and Baptista 1988). The large water birds could not molt sequentially because if these birds, which have heavy bodies and relatively small wings, lose even one primary feather they have trouble flying. Therefore, large water birds will find a secluded place with plenty of food and shelter from predators, and will molt there. Ducks have two molts a year; one molt is functional and one molt is to get a new set of attractive feathers to lure a mate. Geese, on the other hand, just molt once a year. Molting does not occur in the season when the ducks and geese are to fly south for the winter, whether they end up actually migrating or not.

Could the questioned feather be from feathers that happened to be on a road, any road that the car drove on? Could the driver of the vehicle have hit a duck or goose and that is how the down happened to be in the engine block of the car? The large water birds in the area would have molted long before November so the chance of down floating around, which is light and fluffy and easily blown by the wind, is unlikely. Down would have been stuck to some vegetation long before November.[2]

[2] The author experienced a serendipitous event during this investigation. She hit a duck with her car. Purely an accident; however, no down was found in the radiator of the author's car. When something on the ground is hit, like a duck, most of the debris will go under the car and to the rear. A bird would have to be hit "on the wing" to get any down on the radiator. This was not attempted by the author.

(a)

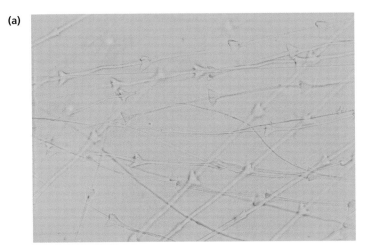

Figure 8.9

*Triangular nodes from
(a) a duck (400×), and
(b) a parakeet (400×)*

(b)

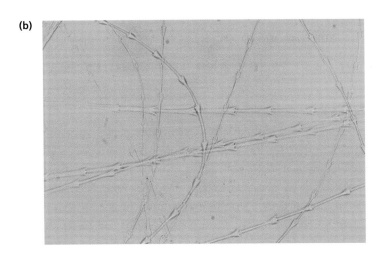

The evidence in this case was a piece of down, not the downy barbules from a contour feather. Fortunately the node structure was present and apparent in the piece of down recovered from the radiator of Portas's car. Comparing the evidential down with that of down from the victim's jacket and that of down recovered from a known source (a live duck) something else became apparent. The known down from the duck was very dirty and sticky. This material is why down is washed several times for use in clothing or bedding. The evidential down (from the car), even though it was stuck in the radiator, was still clean and not sticky to the touch, much like the down recovered from the victim's jacket. Therefore, it could be concluded that the down from the radiator was not from a natural source but had been processed for use in a garment or textile.

Figure 8.10
Quadrilobed nodes from a dove (400×).

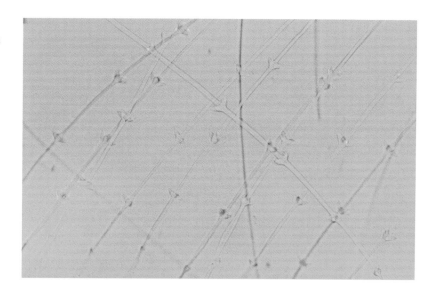

THE TESTIMONY AND THE VERDICT

Almost a year after the victim's body was found, Nicholas Cortez and Franco Portas went on trial for murder in the first degree. Montoya relayed his version of what happened the night of November 8, including the part about the knife, the part that he left out of the first two interviews he had with the local detectives.

All of the forensic evidence was presented. The testimony regarding the down started with a simple explanation of the structure of down, the barbs, barbules, and nodes. Photomicrographs of both the questioned down recovered from the car and the known down from the victim's jacket were shown to the jury, describing the triangular nodes and how they are common to waterfowl and to parrots.

The jury came back with a verdict of guilty for murder in the first degree for both Nicholas Cortez and Franco Portas. The case for Cortez is currently on appeal.

SUMMARY

In the closing arguments of this case, the defense attorneys attempted to negate the blood evidence by referring to Franco Portas's version of events, testimony regarding the jeans and how these were out of the defendant's possession while Montoya made the drug deal. They also tried to impeach Montoya's testimony citing inconsistencies in his statements and also citing the fact that he had lied to the local police twice before telling them the truth. There was no dispute, however, that the two defendants were in the Lincoln together. Could the trace evidence in the form of one piece of down recovered from that vehicle have tipped the scales and swayed the jury?

REFERENCES

Chandler, A.C. (1916) *A Study of the Structure of Feathers, with Reference to their Taxonomic Significance*, Publications in Zoology, N13, V11, Berkeley, CA: University of California.

Day, M.G. (1966) *J. Zoology*, 148, 201–217.

Deedrick, D.W. and Mullery, J.P. (1981) "Feathers are not lightweight evidence," *FBI Law Enforcement Bulletin* 50(9), 22–23.

Robertson, J., Harkin, C. and Govan, J. (1982) *J. For. Sci. Soc.*, V24, 85–98.

Welty, J.C. and Baptista, L.F. (1988) *The Life of Birds*, 4th edn, New York, NY: Saunders College Publications.

Wood, N.A. (1951) *The Birds of Michigan*, Ann Arbor: University of Michigan Press.

CHAPTER 9

A CASE OF CROSS-TRANSFER

Max M. Houck

INTRODUCTION

On March 4, 1998, at about 10 minutes past 5.00 p.m., Joyce Morgan[1] arrived home to find her house had been broken into and ransacked. The county Sheriff's office was called and a deputy dispatched. A cursory walk through the house revealed numerous items missing and the house in disarray but Morgan's real concern was for her daughter, Alice. Normally, Alice would arrive home at 3.00 p.m. from school, change clothes, and take care of her 4-H animals. She was instructed not to answer the phone unless she recognized the voice once the answering machine picked up or to answer the door unless it was someone she knew or a neighbor. During the brief walk-through, Alice was nowhere to be seen.

Additional deputies and crime scene technicians were called to properly process the house and its contents. Morgan told the deputies that when she arrived home, she knocked on the door for Alice to come out. Hearing no reply or movement from within, Morgan went back to her car to retrieve her keys. Seeing her house had been burgled, she quickly ran through the rooms looking for Alice, finally exiting the rear door. Morgan saw her neighbor, Harold Adams, running across her backyard carrying something. Adams was known in the neighborhood as an argumentative drug addict who had been arrested previously for minor infractions. Morgan yelled at Adams about being on her property; the neighbors had been in disputes over an adjacent fence between their properties. Adams ran through a hole in the fence into his yard. Morgan says she called, "Where's my daughter?," to which Adams replied, "I didn't do it! I didn't do it!"

Morgan gave the officers a quick list of items that had been stolen, although she conceded there would undoubtedly be more. Odd things had been taken, some of which were found in the yard outside of Morgan's home: a trunk, a pie plate, an answering machine, plastic water containers, cans of beer from the refrigerator, and a black guitar case, among others. No sign of forced entry was evident. Deputies and investigators went to Adams's house to ask him about the burglary.

[1] All names have been changed.

Adams was a familiar figure to the police. He had been in trouble with the law for things like failing to pay taxi drivers, theft, weapons possessions and other infractions. He had been convicted three times, in 1980 of second degree burglary and receiving stolen property and in 1984 of second degree burglary while armed with a firearm; his most recent conviction, in 1990, was for possessing controlled substances. Adams had also attempted to rob a store but was shot by the retailer, apprehended, and served two years. The neighbors also knew Adams, and avoided him. He was known locally as a drunk, a drug addict, and an oddball. According to neighbors, Adams and his mother argued constantly and Adams had a quick and nasty temper. Adams had lived in the trailer behind his mother's house for many years but she had tried to evict him for the last 10 years or so. Adams had moved into the house when Mrs Adams broke her hip and was hospitalized. Living alone, on disability, and alternating between a drug habit and the methadone clinic, Adams had not paid the utilities in months.

The Adams house was dark and locked. The officers asked Adams if they could come in to ask him questions about Alice. Adams consented to a search of his house and the trailer on his property. Adams's story was that he had seen a Mexican in the Morgan's yard and had gone to investigate. While checking on the Morgans' house, Adams said he knocked on the door and Alice had answered. Adams made sure she was alright and asked her for a glass of water. When he gave the glass back to Alice, Adams said he became dizzy and fell. Alice caught him and he returned to his house.

This story didn't sit well with the investigators for several reasons. A couple of Mexicans had been seen in the neighborhood recently, but none of the neighbors questioned thought they were a threat; the men had merely been looking for odd jobs. Adams maintained that the Mexicans had attempted to rob a neighbor, although the neighbor said this was false. No other neighbors recalled seeing any strangers in the neighborhood that day. Adams would not normally visit the Morgan house. Alice was much smaller than Adams and could have hardly born his weight had he fallen. An interview with a neighbor yielded the following information. At about 3.30 p.m., Adams had knocked on the door of Richard Bradley looking for cigarettes. Bradley sold him a spare pack for $1. Bradley said that Adams appeared "nervous and was not acting normal." Adams carried a fractured walking stick, and he showed it to Bradley, saying he had broken it by hitting a Mexican the previous night. Mrs Bradley, who had been a drug counselor and was familiar with the behavior of people under the influence, said that Adams was "wired to the gills . . . he looked like he was doing speedballs[2] or something." Bradley noticed that, in addition to the walking stick, Adams was carrying a butcher knife and a piece of bamboo in the front waistband of his pants. Mrs Bradley then asked Mr Bradley to make Adams leave.

[2] "Speedballs" or "speed-balling" refers to combining heroin and methamphetamine or cocaine.

Other evidence was mounting against Adams: a stereo speaker, a cordless telephone, an answering machine and other items were found in his back yard; jewelry, with apparent bloodstains, was found in his bathroom that was identified as being from the Morgan house; and, significantly, a can of beer. A sheriff's deputy noted that the beer was the same brand as was missing from the Morgan's refrigerator. He touched the can: it was "ice cold." This struck the officer as odd, since the electricity to Adams's house had been turned off for some time and no ice chests were in sight.

Adams was asked to come to the sheriff's office to make an official statement and he agreed. While sitting in the police cruiser smoking a cigarette, Adams heard Joyce Morgan begin shrieking and crying loudly. No one said anything, except Adams, who casually asked the deputies, "Oh, did they find her?"

THE CRIME SCENE

Meanwhile, the Morgan house and the surrounding property was being systematically searched, photographed and sketched as a crime scene (Figure 9.1). A search team and tracking dogs had been requested to look for Alice; the FBI was notified as is typical in potential kidnappings. Neighbors were questioned about that afternoon and the usual habits of Morgan, her daughter, and Adams. A neighbor recalled seeing Alice and a schoolmate walking from the bus at about 3.00 p.m. It was now much later and there was no sign of her.

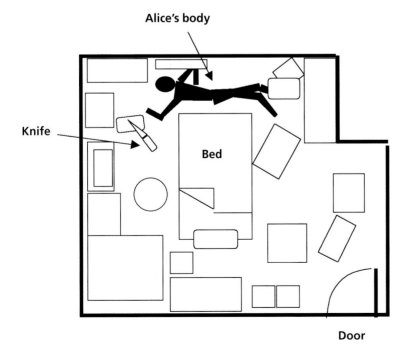

Figure 9.1
Crime scene sketch.

Figure 9.2
Victim's bedroom.

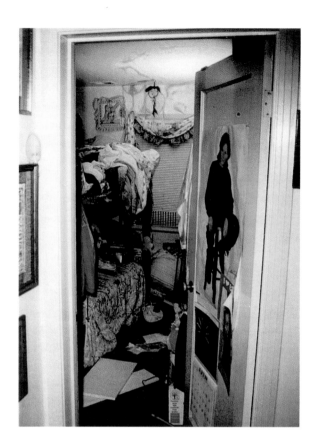

Two investigators conducted a thorough walk-through to confirm that Alice was not in the house. They found her in her cramped, furniture-filled bedroom (Figure 9.2) behind the bed. She had been beaten and her throat had been cut twice (Figure 9.3). Her body had been obscured by the clutter in the room; she had been lying there, dead, the entire time.

The autopsy showed a massive array of wounds, abrasions, cuts:

- a cluster of at least seven lacerations of the right frontal and parietal scalp,
- confluent contusions of the right frontal and temporal scalp extending down into the right eye and cheek,
- bruises and abrasions on her right ear, elbow, wrist and hand, as well as her lip, chin and back,
- a comminuted fracture on the rear of her skull that cracked it all the way to her eyes, and
- a gaping incised wound 4″ in length across her throat, severing her right common carotid artery and right internal jugular vein and perforating her esophagus; visible in the depths of this wound was the broken end of a knife blade, attesting to the force of the attack.

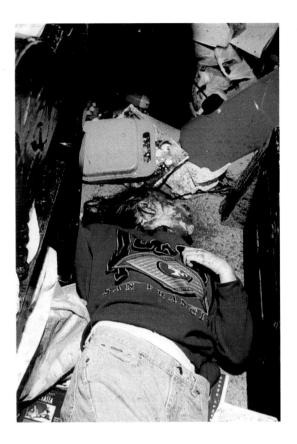

Figure 9.3
Victim as she was found.

The pathologist's opinion was that Alice had died from multiple head and neck injuries and that it would have taken her several minutes to die.

The State's prosecutor assigned to the case wrote a letter to the FBI Laboratory requesting analysis of the evidence. The attorney apologized throughout the letter for the amount of evidence submitted but knew that any minute amount of evidence could be crucial to the prosecution of the case. DNA analysis was being conducted by the State's crime laboratory but the trace evidence was submitted to the FBI Laboratory because, according to the attorney, the State lab lacked the expertise to perform hair comparisons. The subject's and the victim's clothing worn at the time of the crime had not been, and would not be, processed for trace evidence. The crime had shocked the small rural community and the State's Attorney would seek the death penalty. The FBI Laboratory was the attorney's only feasible hope for trace analysis.

ANALYSIS

The submitted items were inventoried, labeled, and described. The list of specimens included:

- paper toweling from the suspect's residence;
- debris from the adjoining fence;
- bags used to cover the victim's hands;
- debris from the victim's hands;
- items from the victim, including fingernail clippings, sweatshirt, shoes, and shirt;
- items from the suspect, including poncho and shirt;
- known hair samples from the victim, suspect, the victim's mother, victim's mother's boyfriend, suspect's girlfriend, assorted pets in the house;
- known carpet samples from the victim's house;
- known fiber samples from various dolls and stuffed animals in the victim's room.

Despite the attorney's concern, no more than about 40 items were ultimately submitted for analysis. Often, crime scene personnel in a desperate attempt not to make a mistake nevertheless err on the side of caution and collect many, many items of evidence. Most of these do nothing more than create a glut of evidence in the laboratory and a backlog of cases for the examiner. No one can deny that thoroughness is the watchword for crime scene processing but thoughtfulness is nearly as important. Blindly grabbing every item of clothing from a suspect's or victim's closet with no regard as to *why* those items are being collected does a disservice to the laboratory and, eventually, to the investigator as well. Given the intense media coverage that can smother a breaking case, the fear of later scrutiny and blame at not having collected every possible item of evidence can be understood, if not appreciated. But fear is a poor justification, and reason, tempered by the circumstances of the crime and experience, should dictate what is collected.

Sampling as evidence collection is not a statistical approach but does involve the use of random, judgment and bulk sampling techniques. Sampling a population is a basic concept in science. It is rarely possible to collect, identify and examine an entire population. This is particularly true of forensic science due to concerns of the time-line of events in a crime, contact between those involved, and contamination. Sampling occurs during the collection of evidence at the crime scene and its subsequent processing in the laboratory. Trace evidence, by its nature, requires utilizing samples from larger populations to characterize and compare trace materials. Robertson (1992) states that while it is not possible to collect everything, the crime scene technician must make informed decisions about what to retrieve. Regarding fibers, he makes the point that it is important to "ensur[e] that adequate and *representative* known and control samples have been taken" [p. 44; emphasis added]. "Representative" is not used here in any specific statistical meaning but merely to denote that a suitable and adequate sample was taken from the total population of hairs and fibers present.

This concept extends into the laboratory. Debris from the evidence may consist of numerous hairs and fibers, some from the item itself, some from contact the wearer has made with other people, places or objects. Examining a subset of these populations of fibers is the only practical method in forensic casework. As Robertson points out,

> Other than in exceptional circumstances it is quite ludicrous to expect that it would be practical, or serve any useful purpose, to attempt to determine the origin of all the extraneous fibres found to be present [p. 57].

For example, Gaudette (1988) notes that in one case, over 600 fibers consisting of at least 56 distinct types and colors were removed from one pair of shoes. Sampling, therefore, is the only answer. Addressing the 'how' of sampling, the Scientific Working Group for Materials Analysis (SWGMAT) Fiber Subgroup in Chapter 1, Section 6.0, "Sample Handling," of the *Forensic Fiber Examination Guidelines* lists three basic types of sampling:

- *probability sampling* (so-called "random sampling"), in which every unit in the population has a known, non-zero probability of being included in the sample (e.g. collecting about 33 per cent of the fibers from a pillbox or a taping and mounting them).
- *nonprobability* or *judgment sampling*, in which every unit in the population either is or is not included in the sample based upon certain characteristics it has in common with other units of interest (e.g. mounting only red trilobal carpet-type fibers from the victim's evidence given the suspect has red carpet as a possible source).
- *bulk* or *lot sampling*, in which a sampling unit is taken from a larger amount of material that does not consist of discrete, identifiable units. Special considerations are involved with bulk sampling, such as where the sample is taken, how much sample is taken and if the sample is considered representative of the lot (e.g. cutting a swatch from a garment for fabric and fiber examination).

The context of the crime and the item determine what constitutes a proper, adequate or "representative" sample. The SWGMAT Fiber Subgroup has determined that "[s]amples are adequate for analysis" when,

> they are taken in a manner consistent with generally recognized and accepted sampling techniques and practices within the context of the proposed analyses. All of the above sampling methods have their place, and one may be more feasible than another, given crime scene or laboratory constraints. The examiner must be able to explain how the samples were taken and why that procedure was used [p. 6].

While other forensic laboratories may not use the same terms listed above, they nonetheless employ similar methods of sampling.

A variety of methods are used to collect fibrous evidence, including picking with tweezers, taping, scraping, and vacuuming. All of these methods sample the population of hairs and fibers from an object, although in different ways. In this sense, *all evidence collection is sampling* and every trace evidence examiner samples during the course of his or her casework. Even if a taping is searched for hairs or fibers, those hairs or fibers chosen are a sample of the total collected.

Many forensic laboratories, particularly in Europe, select target fibers from known samples and then search for these fibers on questioned items. Some laboratories, including the FBI's, also search a sample of the debris removed from the evidence for fibers that may be held in common between a suspect, victim and/or crime scene. Employing only target fibers precludes this type of examination and could be detrimental to an investigation, particularly in terms of lead value. These so-called "common" fibers (because they are common between the two items, not because they are common in the population of all fibers) can provide useful information about items that may have been used or encountered during the commission of a crime but are not currently available (see Chapter 6).

All or part of the debris from a specimen is mounted on glass microscope slides and may be termed a "representative sample." The term "representative" is used because this sample, in some way, represents the population of hairs or fibers recovered from the item of evidence. The representative sample is not intended to be a 20 per cent sample without replacement, for example: it merely contains an intentional or random subset of the collected debris. The concept of a representative sample in the non-statistical sense is common in trace evidence. Bisbing (1982) notes that "[e]xemplary hairs from each body region must be *representative* of that part of the body" [p. 207; emphasis added]. In fact, he suggests the use of the stereomicroscope to obtain

> a rapid overview of the range of characteristics associated with the hairs. The examiner can then judiciously select hairs *representative* of the exemplar's characteristics for more detailed examinations. [p. 208; emphasis added]

Sampling occurs unintentionally when fibers are found to be in common between suspect and victim as the examiner has no idea that such fibers exist prior to examination. The representative sample is searched microscopically for hairs, target fibers, and/or fibers in common. These questioned materials are then compared with known samples. The collected debris in the pillbox is available if, for any reason, the examiner wishes to go back and review it.

The use of sampling is central to the examination of trace evidence. The number of hairs and fibers collected at any single crime scene can very quickly total in the hundreds, if not thousands. A subset or sample of hairs and fibers that are collected from evidence are examined as a matter of necessity. One or more methods of sampling may be employed based upon the context of the crime, the evidence that is submitted and the observations of the technician and examiner. No strict or even informal statistical approaches are used in this process. A sample is adequate if it presents the information required to accept or reject the investigative hypothesis proposed. The term "representative" is used to indicate that a subset of the collected debris has been mounted on a glass microscope slide and that additional debris remains in the pillbox container.

Care must be taken with sampling such that unconscious biases do not creep into a procedure. While target samples, that is, samples from the population of interest, are important to identify, they can blind investigators to the possibilities afforded by the available evidence. Quota sampling, where there is a fixed number of samples each of which has to fall within certain predetermined values, should probably be avoided in forensic science. This was, incidentally, one of the downfalls of the Dewey/Truman election predictions that are infamous to students of statistics and polling (Wild and Seber 2000). Quotas have no place in forensic science sampling and casework.

The validity of the samples taken is predicated on the proper questions being asked. If you select a sampling regime based on the questions you want answered without regard for the way in which the questions are worded (that is, bias), you will end up with very different questions. For example, a survey was carried out at a university to study the way in which wording affects responses. Two versions of a questionnaire were prepared that were the same except for two questions. The first version asked:

1. Are you in favor of giving special priority to buses in the rush hour?
2. Do you think that the cost of catching a bus into (the) university is too high?

The questions were worded differently in version 2:

1. Are you in favor of giving special priority to buses in the rush hour, or should cars have just as much priority as buses?
2. Taking into account the problems and costs associated with parking, do you think that the cost of catching a bus into (the) university is too high?

The two versions were distributed randomly amongst 1154 students; 585 responded to the first version and 569 responded to version two. For the first question, 68 per cent replied yes to version 1 and 47 per cent to version 2; but

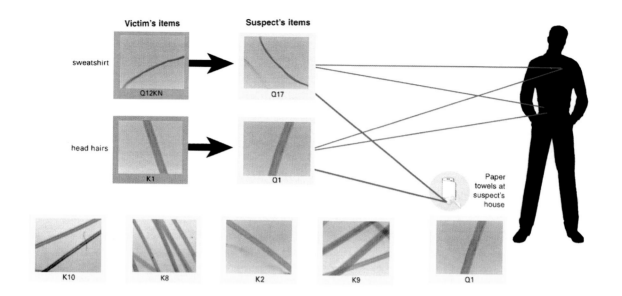

Figure 9.4

Transfer of trace evidence from subject to victim.

with question 2, 75 per cent said yes to version 1 and 63 per cent to version 2. The results differ depending on what sides of an issue are offered and different wordings lead to different responses (Wild and Seber 2000). One can easily see how the questions posed, and possibly presumed, by an investigator or an examiner could lead to a loss of data through ignorance or assumption. Wording is just as important in evidence interpretation as it is in framing the initial questions.

Returning to our case, the smaller items such as the fingernails were examined under a stereomicroscope and any debris was removed with tweezers and mounted on glass microscope slides. The larger items, such as clothing, were processed in special rooms at the FBI Laboratory. These rooms contain racks for holding large items above a table. Clean paper is placed beneath the items and changed between items. The items are then gently scraped with a large metal spatula to dislodge the debris. The debris collects on the paper and is then transferred to a small plastic lidded container called a pillbox. The quality assurance procedures involved with scraping are different than with other collection methods and it requires a meticulous approach to cleaning the processing room and its contents before and after each use. Protective clothing is also required. While scraping is not performed by some laboratories, it is a very effective and efficient collection technique where large items or a large number of items must be processed.

The results of the analysis correlated with the terrible evidence from the autopsy: Alice's last moments had been violent but she had not died without a struggle. There was a number of cross-transfers of hairs and fibers from a variety

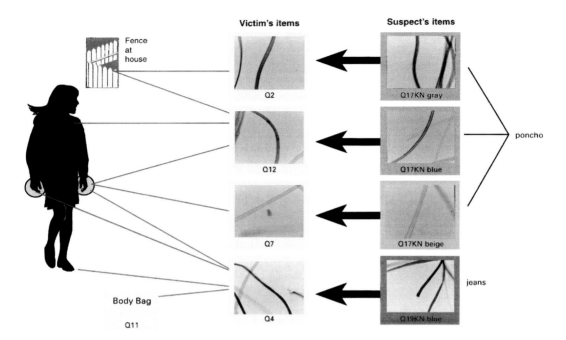

Victim's items   Suspect's items

Fence at house

Q2   Q17KN gray

Q12   Q17KN blue

poncho

Q7   Q17KN beige

Body Bag

Q11   Q4   Q19KN blue   jeans

of sources intimate to both Alice and Adams. Blue, gray, and beige polyester fibers were found on Alice's sweatshirt, on her hands and under her fingernails. These fibers had the same microscopic and optical properties as the known blue, gray, and beige polyester fibers from Adam's poncho (Figure 9.4). The poncho was made up of a large number of fiber types and readily shed many fibers. Some of the blue and gray polyester fibers were found on the fence at the gap between the two yards.

Blue rayon fibers were found on Alice's hands, under her fingernails, and on her shoes. These rayon fibers were distinctive in that they were dyed very darkly and had pigmentation on their surface. These fibers had the same microscopic and optical properties as known rayon fibers from Adams's jeans. These jeans, made under the label of Roglins Stretch Jeans, were composed of 43 per cent cotton, 29 per cent rayon, and 28 per cent polyester. Normally, blue jeans are 100 per cent cotton and, because they are almost all dyed with natural or synthetic indigo dyes which fade differentially with wear, are considered to have little forensic value (Grieve 1990). The evidentiary value of these jeans is notable simply because of their composition and that they shed not the cotton fibers but the rayon. More of these fibers were found on the body bag used to transport Alice to the morgue, a product of secondary transfer.

Red cotton fibers were found on Adams's poncho and his shirt. These fibers exhibited the same microscopic and optical properties as known red cotton fibers from Alice's sweatshirt (Figure 9.5). More of these red cotton fibers were found on paper towels at Adams's house in the bathroom trashcan.

All of the fibers in this case were examined by comparison microscopy, polarized light microscopy, fluorescent microscopy, chemical solubility, and microspectrophotometry in the visible range of light.

Brown Caucasian head hairs with the same microscopic characteristics as Alice's head hairs were found on Adams's poncho and shirt and on the paper towels in the trashcan. These head hairs were microscopically dissimilar to the other known head hair standards provided by the investigators. While not a means of positive personal identification, microscopic hair comparisons can provide strong associative evidence (Bisbing 1982). The number of hairs that had the same microscopic characteristics as Alice's and that were recovered from different items also added to the significance.

CONCLUSION

The overwhelming number of trace evidence transfers was only a small portion of the evidence presented at Adams's trial. The jury deliberated briefly, returning a verdict of guilty in less than three hours.

REFERENCES

Bisbing, R.E. (1982) "The forensic identification and association of human hair," in *Forensic Science Handbook*, Vol. 1, ed. R. Saferstein, Englewood Cliffs, NJ: Prentice Hall.

Gaudette, B.D. (1988) "The forensic aspects of textile fibre examination," in *Forensic Science Handbook*, Vol. 2, ed. R. Saferstein, Englewood Cliffs, NJ: Prentice Hall.

Grieve, M.C. (1990) "Fibres and their examination in forensic science," in *Forensic Science Progress*, Vol. 4, eds A. Maehly and R.L. Williams, Berlin, Germany: Springer-Verlag.

Robertson, J. (ed.) (1992) *The Forensic Examination of Fibres*, New York, NY: Ellis Horwood.

Scientific Working Group for Materials Analysis (1999) *Forensic Fiber Examination Guidelines.*

Scientific Working Group for Materials Analysis (1999) *Trace Evidence Recovery Guidelines.*

Wild, C.J. and Seber, G.A.F. (2000) *Chance Encounters*, New York: John Wiley and Sons.

AUTHOR INDEX